no i will

By

Richard Matthews

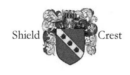

Shield Crest

© Copyright 2018 Richard Matthews

All rights reserved

ISBN: 978-1-912505-24-1

MMXVIII

A CIP catalogue record for this book
is available from the British Library

Published by
ShieldCrest Publishing Ltd.,
Aylesbury, Buckinghamshire,
HP18 0TF England
Tel: +44 (0) 333 8000 890
www.shieldcrest.co.uk

Dedication

This book is dedicated to the amazing women who have blessed and shaped my life.

For Julie, thank you for being quite simply, the best wife in the world.

For Emily, who never once complained that her brother took up a greater share of our time and for not hesitating for a second to give her blessing to me writing this book.

For my mum, for everything, you are truly amazing.

For June, my mother-in-law, I only wish I had half your energy, you are a legend.

And finally, to Susan Favre who gave us a home in her beautiful village, I will be forever in your debt, may you rest in peace.

Author Biography

Richard Matthews was born in Brighton in 1971 but spent the majority of his childhood while growing up in Wimborne, Dorset. His parents, Dudley and Diana were publicans and he has two brothers, Steve and Pete and a sister Sally.

For the past sixteen years he has lived in a small picturesque village called Chettle with his wife Julie where they raised their twins, William and Emily.

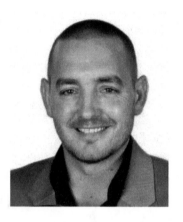

This is Richard's first book and is a very honest account of his experiences raising his son who has special needs, a roller coaster of tears and frustrations followed by laughter and pure joy.

Richard's motivation for writing this book was to help shine a light on the difficulties parents in similar situations face on a daily basis but ultimately to give hope.

Raising a special child has been the toughest challenge of his life but without doubt, the most rewarding too.

Contents

Chapter One

Cartwheels Down The Corridors

July 1996

I stepped out of the shower and had to grab the side as a massive wave of nausea hit me. My first thought was, *Julie's pregnant.* I smiled to myself, and dismissed the thought just as quickly; there was no reason to suspect she was pregnant and, besides, men don't get morning sickness! The nausea passed as soon as it had arrived and I didn't give it another thought until three hours later when Julie phoned me at work and said she needed to come in and see me. They say your life can change in a moment, and I knew then that mine had.

The hour or so before she turned up at the garage seemed to last forever. The garage was a car showroom in Poole that I had opened two years before, when I was twenty-three. I had never had any particular interest in cars, but at eighteen I got a job as a car salesman and, after five years, I took a risk and opened my own showroom. I paced around the forecourt trying to convince myself I couldn't possibly know and that it could be any number of things. When she walked in, if I'd had any doubt about what she had to tell me it disappeared in that moment, as she looked so worried but somehow more beautiful than ever. Julie was a really pretty girl with dark brown eyes, long dark hair and an amazing body; she was also one of the kindest, most caring people I'd ever met. I can't remember the exact words she stumbled over, through tears, but I held her and told her how much I loved her and that everything would be fine.

We had only been seeing each other for six months – she was my sister's best friend and they shared a rented flat just around the corner from mine. Although we were very much in love, a baby was

1

definitely not on the agenda. Julie was only twenty-one, and she worked Monday to Friday as a nanny for a young girl and spent most weekends clubbing in Bournemouth. When I wasn't working I was riding fast motorbikes and throwing trouble-makers out of my brother's pub. I was running my own business, but I certainly wasn't getting rich as there was no consistency to the motor trade. It was feast or famine, and mostly famine. The reality of the situation started to dawn on me: I would have to provide for a family and life was never going to be the same again.

A couple of weeks later I was sitting in my office watching the heavens open, soaking the twenty cars I had just finished cleaning, when Julie phoned. She was bleeding heavily and sobbing her heart out, and my world came crashing down. My beautiful girl was frightened and in pain and we were losing our baby. The pain was unbearable. I felt utterly devastated and helpless. I had never felt grief like it. A waking nightmare taking place in slow motion. I was on my own at work and desperately worried when a friend called in for a coffee. He saw the state I was in and said he would keep an eye on the cars so I could go and see Julie. I called her on the way and told her we were going to hospital. I couldn't believe how poorly Julie looked, as white as a sheet and in terrible pain. We managed to get an emergency scan at Poole Hospital, and I drove us there in a kind of terrified silence, dreading having our worst fears confirmed.

I remember the sonographer lifting Julie's shirt to put the ultrasound to her tummy and feeling like we didn't belong there. She looked so young, and had a washboard stomach, she couldn't possibly be having a baby. After what seemed like an age he said he couldn't hear a heartbeat, but not to let that worry us as she was only five weeks gone, it could be just too faint to hear. We were told to make sure Julie got lots of rest and to come back in two weeks' time for another scan. How the hell were we going to last two weeks feeling like this?

We were so worried, and by the end of the day were both emotionally drained, so I took Julie back to my flat to sleep. I owned a converted malthouse in the heart of Wimborne, Dorset. It was the ultimate bachelor pad, on the top floor, with views over the Minster Church, a huge lounge with exposed beams, and a spiral staircase leading up to the second bedroom. I shared it with my dog Henry, a black Labrador I'd had from a puppy. We were inseparable and he came to work with me every day. He was an amazing, intelligent dog, and you could tell he knew something was wrong as he kept sniffing Julie's tummy and his eyes were sad. I cuddled up to Julie and hoped that when we woke up this would all have been a nightmare.

The next morning Julie looked a little better; some colour had returned to her face and the pain had subsided. We spent the next two weeks just hoping that our baby would be alright. It felt like the longest two weeks of my life. The day of the scan arrived and, for the second time in as many weeks, we were sitting in a waiting room surrounded by very large, heavily pregnant women – and there was Julie in a pencil-skirt and crop-top revealing a flat, toned stomach. Every now and again a husband would steal a glance, only to get a nudge or an angry stare from their wife. We were called in and for the second time Julie climbed up on the bed and had that gel stuff smeared over her stomach and the sonographer started to move his ultrasound tool around in circular motions. Time seemed to stand still. I was so nervous, but I managed a reassuring look at Julie. Then the sonographer stopped moving his hand and said the words that would change our lives forever:

"Is there any history of twins in your family?"

My heart started to race and my mouth went dry. Julie tried to explain that her mum thought she had miscarried, but was still carrying Julie, so perhaps she had been a twin and that my dad was a twin. She was speaking at a million miles an hour, but I was just hearing noise. I just wanted him to finish what he was saying.

"Well, congratulations, you two, you are having twins and the heartbeats are very strong."

Julie turned around to face me with the biggest smile on her face and tears in her eyes – and then her expression changed as she remembered what I'd said on the way to hospital.

"Please don't do cartwheels," she said, somewhat embarrassed.

3

Ever since I was a young boy I'd been convinced that I would have twins – identical twin boys, just like my dad and his brother Neil. I'd grown up with so much admiration for them both; they were big strong men and fiercely competitive but also so very close. Whether they were golfing, fishing, playing cards or snooker, they would compete as if their lives depended on it. You could guarantee when my dad phoned Neil it would be engaged as Neil was trying to call him. They even broke the same arm at the same time while miles apart, so I was always fascinated by the apparent twin telepathy. My uncle Neil died tragically, aged just forty-seven. I wanted twins so badly that I had told Julie on the way to the hospital that if it was twins I would do cartwheels down the corridors. She needn't have been embarrassed. She had no idea how good my cartwheels were!

I remember looking at Julie, all seven stone of her and wondering how on earth she was ever going to fit one baby in, let alone two. I was the happiest man alive, and I told her what an amazing mummy she'd be. She had studied childcare and child psychology at college and was incredible with children, so kind and caring, with unlimited patience. We left the hospital and set off to tell everyone our news.

Julie's parents Ron and June were quiet, country folk. They lived in an idyllic village called Chettle, in between Blandford and Salisbury, and grew strawberries and tended the ground. Ron was not a big man but when his sleeves were rolled up you could see the strength in his arms from a lifetime of manual work. June was attractive, and in great shape, but she had no time for make-up or visits to a salon. She lived in jeans and wellies, and the two of them reminded me of Tom and Barbara from *The Good Life*. They had no interest in money or material things, but were the two most content people I'd ever met. Like my parents they were hard workers, and very much in love, but that was where the similarities ended. My mum and dad, Dudley and Diana, were publicans, loud and confident, and the throwers of the best parties around. My mum was the life and soul and, despite raising four children and working long hours, she always looked beautiful; in fact, she bore a striking resemblance to the princess of the same name. My dad was a big guy. He looked like a cross between Tom Selleck and Sean Connery. He was a great story teller, and very popular, but you wouldn't want to get on the wrong side of him. Fortunately, although Julie and I were not married, both our parents were really happy for us.

On 10th March 1997, Julie turned twenty-two, and was now thirty-nine weeks pregnant and apparently three weeks late. We had no idea that it was unusual for twins to go full term. We had attended all the scans; however, we hadn't attended any antenatal classes, and it transpired we should have had regular appointments with the consultant too. I'm not sure how we slipped through the net with the consultant, but not attending antenatal classes was down to us. I was working sixty-hour weeks and really had no interest in sitting around holding hands learning how to breathe in and out. June reminded us that her sheep gave birth out in the fields on their own without any classes, so we would be fine too! I loved her down-to-earth, matter-of-fact attitude, and it got me off the hook. The reality, though, was the twins needed to come out and they obviously were in no hurry to do so on their own. An appointment was made for the following day for Julie to go into hospital and be induced. We went out that evening, on her birthday, for a Chinese meal – we'd been told spicy food and sex can help bring on the labour and, obviously not one to stand in the way of progress, I duly obliged. I think the only thing it produced was heartburn but it was fun trying!

I genuinely thought that the following evening we would go to hospital, Julie would be induced, and would then give birth. I was surprised when the nurses told me to go home and get a good night's sleep as nothing would happen that night.

The next morning, Julie phoned at around seven o'clock and asked me to come back to the hospital. She was lonely and had been pacing the corridors for most of the night in pain and now just wanted me back. I got up and showered and then heard the phone ringing again.

"Hello, Mr Matthews, this is the midwife. Julie has just been taken into the labour ward so could you get down here as soon as you can?"

I said that couldn't be possible as I'd only spoken to her ten minutes before! But I was assured that this was it and the birth of the twins was imminent. 'Get here safely but get here quickly' was the advice. I went into full Benny Hill mode, doing everything at a hundred miles an hour. The journey to Poole Hospital from Wimborne should take about fifteen minutes, but I drove like a lunatic, swearing at every slow car and, with my hand permanently on the horn, I managed it in less than ten. I parked the car and ran as fast as I could, jumping whole staircases with one leap, and sliding round the corridors nearly flattening a few people on the way. I made it . . . with just the fourteen hours to spare!

Now I am sure that when some men tell you the day their child was born was the best day of their life they mean it; for me, though, it was a day spent completing crosswords and word searches and endless walks to and from various vending machines. Julie had been given an epidural for pain relief so there were no dramas, no holding her hand and wiping her brow, or getting sworn at while telling her everything would be okay, just hour after hour of waiting. Eventually it was decided that the twins were not going to come out on their own and Julie would have to have a caesarean. It was disappointing, but we had been warned to expect it. I was given a gown and a mask, and very quickly everyone seemed ready for surgery. After the slowest day of my life suddenly people were moving like they were trying to catch a plane!

I just had time to make one final phone call to my parent's house to give them the latest news. Since lunchtime they'd had a houseful – my brothers and sister and loads of our friends all drinking and celebrating and waiting for my call, I could hear them all partying and I was looking forward to joining them later. There was a book running on the twins, boys or girls, weights and time of birth. We had decided from the start we did not want to know the sex. I, of course, was convinced they were identical boys, but everyone had their own beliefs, whether it was based on the shape of Julie's tummy or the ring test. I had never seen a pregnant tummy like it. From behind Julie was still tiny, as she hadn't gained weight anywhere else, but you'd see her tummy about two minutes before she came around a bend. It was like a cartoon belly and the skin was so stretched it was almost transparent. We had decided on names for the twins, William and James for the boys, and Emily and Jessica for the girls; there was no reason behind the choices other than they were just favourites we both agreed on.

At nine-thirty pm on Wednesday 12th March 1997, William Dudley Matthews was born. He weighed five pounds and seven ounces and needed a helping hand to catch his first breath and find his voice: a slap on the foot. And as he was turned upside down we heard his first scream. Immediately the attention switched to the next one, and I waited for his brother to be delivered, only this time the doctor looked up, and with a comment about how clever we were he delivered our baby girl. Emily Kay Matthews was born just one minute later and weighed an ounce-and-a-half more.

For the first time in my life I understood unconditional love; I would have given my life in a heartbeat if I could've extended theirs by just a minute, my beautiful gorgeous twins. The feeling of love for them was completely overwhelming. William was tall and slim and looked like a wrinkly old man who'd just done a round with Mike Tyson. It seemed to me as if he'd protected his sister throughout the pregnancy and taken all the stress as a big brother should. I loved him all the more for it. Emily, on the other hand, was the most beautiful baby I'd ever seen, absolute china-doll-perfection, and I remember looking at her for the first time and thinking I'd never been so happy to be wrong. I cuddled Julie and thanked her over and over, and watched with utter amazement as she started to breastfeed our two little miracles. Emily took to it with ease, but William was struggling to latch on – nothing unusual in that, but perhaps just a little sign that, for Will, life would always be more challenging.

The first phone call I made was to Julie's mum. I thought that was the right thing to do, and besides, it would be a relatively quick call. It would be straightforward, to the point, with all the questions asked and answered. June was a very kind-hearted woman, but also a straight-talking country girl. The next call was to my parents and I couldn't wait to break the news. They'd been partying for about eight hours, with a steady flow of friends coming and going. Luckily my mum answered and I'll never forget telling her William and Emily had arrived. The screams were so loud we could've dispensed with the need for a phone. I spent a couple of hours with Julie and the twins, and then headed off to join the now dwindling crowd to celebrate and wet the babies' heads.

I was driving there when it occurred to me to phone Darren and tell him the good news. Darren is my best friend, the first boy I'd met when I joined Wimborne First School aged five and, to this day, forty-one years later, we are still as close as ever. At the time, he was a sergeant in the Royal Marines, and I had no idea where he was in the world. The phone rang forever and just as I was about to hang up I heard a very quiet hello. It turned out he was on exercise in the middle of the Borneo jungle and it was about six in the morning and all the guys were asleep. When I whispered that William and Emily had been born he shouted at the top of his considerable voice, "Get in there, you fucking beauty!" and woke the whole camp up.

With the absence of any alcohol they all celebrated with a bacon and eggs party. I'm not a massive fan of technology but at that moment to be on a mobile talking to my best mate thousands of miles away in the middle of a jungle, sharing that moment, was pretty special.

After celebrating with a few drinks with my family and friends I headed home and climbed into bed – Julie and the twins would be kept in hospital for a few days for observation. I lay in bed tired but elated and unable to sleep and I started to imagine how my children would be. I didn't visualise world leaders or astronauts, Olympians or pop stars, just two people like us but the improved versions. I pictured Emily as beautiful, kind, caring, confident, intelligent and independent. She would ride horses with her mum and head off to the beach with her friends. William would be a big strong man, tough and competitive, with a winner's attitude. He'd be a boxer like me, and my father before, and I wondered at what age he'd be too much for me to handle. He'd play rugby and I'd teach him to play golf and, of course, he'd play off scratch. It was lovely. I was a dad and I was the happiest I'd ever been lying in my bed and willing the hours away so I could get back to see them.

I often wonder how I would have visualised my son's future then if I had known that he had special needs. William is 47XYY, which means he has an extra Y [male] chromosome. It occurs in only 0.1% of the male population and is caused by a random event during the formation of sperm cells. We have twenty-three pairs of chromosomes and the final pair dictates your sex. If you are a girl then your final pair is XX; whereas boys will be XY. Not all, but most boys who have the extra Y chromosome will suffer delays with their development and have learning difficulties. William's problems were very obvious to us but he was nearly five-years-old before he was finally diagnosed.

Raising William has been the biggest challenge of my life, a roller coaster of laughter and pure joy followed by tears and frustrations. We've been through our darkest hours as a family and faced days I wouldn't wish on anyone. I have often been asked if I could turn back the clock, would I roll the dice again? Would I change Will if I could? Not for all the money in the world.

Chapter Two

Life's Most Precious Cargo

William needed a lot of extra care from the nurses on the ward after he was born. He was struggling to feed and was very lethargic so he was placed in an incubator and fed through a tube. It was really tough for us, as we would only get a few hours a day with him and I couldn't help but think, after nine months together, surely this was hard for our twins too. I remember one day a nurse brought him back to the ward and placed him in his clear plastic baby crib next to Emily's. After a little while I picked him up and moved him in to be with Emily. I'm not sure how much credit I can actually take but he definitely improved and Julie and the twins were allowed to come home after five days in hospital.

I will never forget that first journey in the car. It took me bloody ages to work out how to secure the two baby seats and even longer to belt them in. Julie had just been through surgery so couldn't help and she was definitely the practical one. She just smiled and offered advice while I fumbled about like an idiot. The mission was eventually accomplished and we set off for home. I have never driven so slowly in my life. I was carrying life's most precious cargo and it seemed like every car was out to get me and I'm not sure I ever reached twenty miles per hour. If it took me ten minutes to get there the day they were born, I reckon this journey was three times longer. I would've wrapped the whole car in cotton wool if I could.

Those first few months were both magical and exhausting as, in their wisdom, Will and Emily had decided they would feed at different times throughout the night. If we got one hour's sleep without being disturbed it was cause for celebration. As well as running my business, I was selling the flat and trying to find a house. Whilst the flat had been a dream bachelor pad it was up two flights of stairs – not ideal with two of everything to carry. Throughout the pregnancy we would discuss where we wanted to live and every time I thought we'd made a decision Julie would change her mind the next day. I had the estate agent on speed dial, and I honestly thought she was barking mad. It took my mate Darren, who was already a father, to explain to me about hormones. He advised me to just nod my head and agree with her.

We agreed a sale on the flat very quickly, but weren't able to find a house and my parents offered us the opportunity to move in with them rather than lose the sale. I thought we'd only be there for a matter of weeks, but it ended up three months. It's only much later in life I can appreciate what a massive upheaval that must have been for them; like the saying goes, fish and visitors stink after three days! We may have been family, but to share their home with two extra adults and two screaming babies was incredibly generous. We did eventually buy a wonderful house. It was a detached four-bedroomed Edwardian-style property, and all the neighbours were a mixture of dentists, bank managers and head teachers – the kind of last house you own before you downsize. We were by far the youngest couple in the area and it was a massive stretch for me to afford it. Many a time Julie would answer the door and a delivery driver would ask if her mum was in!

We realised when the twins were about six months old that all was not how it should be with William. Julie had a lot of experience working with babies and we, of course, had Emily to compare him to. Emily was very advanced and so naturally people thought there was nothing wrong with William. The general feeling was he was just a lazy boy, and boys develop more slowly than girls. The difference between them was increasing almost on a daily basis, though; like two cars being accelerated at different speeds, the gap kept widening. When you picked Will up for a cuddle he was like a sack of potatoes; he couldn't hold his head up and had very little coordination. Even bottle feeding was a challenge for him. He had a squint and a slight heart murmur, we knew that much; but we were also noticing serious delays with his development.

Most days Julie would drive to Chettle with the twins to see her sister Rachel, who was married to Roland, and had two daughters. Megan was four years old and Rebecca had been born just eight days before the twins. Emily and Rebecca were both walking and talking by nine months; yet Will didn't even crawl until he was eighteen months old. He only had five words for many months. Mum and dad he could say fine, but Emily was 'Umily', Henry was 'Enwy', and hello was 'heyo'. We were getting married on the 14th November 1998 at Chettle Church, when the twins would've been twenty months old, and we were hoping that William would be able to walk down the aisle. Although he had only been crawling for a matter of weeks, he did start to walk about a month before the wedding, using the furniture, his sister or the dog to aid him. The wedding day came and when I turned around and saw my little man in his suit walking on his own down the aisle, I nearly burst with pride. He walked like a Thunderbirds puppet saying heyo to everyone he passed and, as beautiful as Julie looked, he did the unthinkable and upstaged the bride.

We chose to get married in November as it was a quiet time of year for June and my mum. We were going on honeymoon to Thailand for two weeks and our amazing mums had offered to take care of the twins between them. We were extremely lucky, as we desperately needed a holiday. I was under huge amounts of stress with my business, and in the weeks leading up to the wedding, with all that entails, I had to deal with a trading standards investigation, a VAT investigation and ten thousand pounds-worth of vandalism to the cars. Trading standards were looking into an accusation that I'd sold a clocked car. I hadn't. But it was up to me to prove my innocence and the good reputation of the garage was on the line. The VAT investigation was no dawn raid, just my time for a visit from HMRC, but stressful none the less, and fortunately my book-keeping was perfect. Then the vandalism . . . It's just a sad fact that there are idiots out there who do these things; but whilst the repairs were covered by insurance, the loss of earnings weren't.

Having got through all that, and believing the old adage that bad things come in threes, I was just thinking I could relax and look forward to the wedding when my car salesman, Bill, had a heart attack four days before our wedding. He was my only employee, and at fifty-seven he was experienced, reliable and perfectly capable of running the showroom without me for a couple of weeks. He was now in hospital and certainly wouldn't be returning to work for a long time. If I thought I'd known stress before, this was on a whole new level.

For a while it seemed impossible that we would be able to go on honeymoon and I phoned our friends Paddy and Lis to warn them – they were going to move into our house and look after Henry. It transpired that Paddy was not due to start his new job for a few weeks, and as he had worked for me before he could step in and run the garage. So now I was leaving my house, my dog and my business in the hands of my crazy little Irish friend! What could possibly go wrong!

We flew to Phuket the day after the wedding and arrived in the heaviest rain we had ever seen. I had lost thousands of pounds at the garage, had spent thousands more on the wedding and honeymoon and, with all due respect to my friend, I couldn't expect him to earn me anything while I was away. I was consumed with worry and exhausted and we fell into our hotel room and slept for a day! When we finally surfaced, the rain had gone and the sun was shining, and we realised how beautiful the place was. However, after a few days, we were missing the children desperately. Every child we saw reminded us of our children, and we were so close to packing up and leaving early, but a few phone calls home and we were convinced not to.

We started to enjoy ourselves properly, but every time I thought about the garage a black cloud would come over me. I told Julie how I was feeling, and in her very logical, down-to-earth way she said if it made me unhappy I should give it up. I'd never even considered that as a possibility; it was my business and I had to fight to make it work. She was right, though, I could do whatever I wanted, and should do whatever made me happy. She believed in me and trusted that I would always provide no matter what. If I hadn't known it before, this was a shining example of what an incredible girl Julie was and I felt the weight of the world leave my shoulders. After that the honeymoon was amazing. I knew what I was going to do so I relaxed and we had the time of our lives. Soon after returning I did close down the business, and fortunately I had no debts, so after selling most of the stock I was able to make sure Bill was financially secure for the coming months while he recuperated.

What I learned from the experience was what was important. I had so much ambition, and was working ridiculously long hours. I was determined to be successful, but I was missing so much. For ten years in the motor trade I had worked every weekend and bank holiday, only taking a Wednesday afternoon a week off when I would try and squeeze in a game of golf. My time with the children was limited to mornings and evenings for the first two years of their lives and it wasn't enough. I made a decision to change, to work to live and not live to work, to be there as much as possible to raise my children and support Julie. The challenges ahead with William were becoming obvious. Raising any child is tough, but with William you could throw out the rule book.

I was one of four children. My older brother was Steve, my younger brother Pete, and the youngest was my sister Sally. I remember how important it was that we all felt we were treated fairly when we were young, and I'm sure my parents lost count of how many times they heard one of us whine, 'It's not fair'. I remember how hurt I would feel as a child when my immature mind would decide I'd been unfairly treated or been blamed for something that wasn't my fault. The love we all received was, of course, in equal measure; but the reality for all parents is we do treat our children differently, and however much we try to fool ourselves we don't, small differences creep in over time.

I was a very impatient person when the twins were babies and found it extremely stressful just trying to get out of the house when we had to go anywhere. Whenever we went out it felt like we were taking the entire contents of a Boots and Mothercare shop with us. It became a military exercise to try and leave on time and, if you managed it, then that little voice in your head would tell you that you've forgotten something half a mile down the sodding road. At two years old, we could ask Emily to go and get her coat, to make sure she'd been to the toilet, and to put her shoes on – normal stuff to help in the challenge of leaving the house. With William, none of that was possible. If you asked him to go and get his coat you'd inevitably find him some time later sitting on his bed and in a world of his own. He couldn't put his own shoes on, and certainly had no concept of judging when he might need the toilet. So consequently, over time, you realise you are treating them differently, because they have different abilities and needs.

One evening, when the twins were getting ready for bed, I asked them to put their dressing gowns on – they had a pair of pine beds and the dressing gowns were hung over the poles at the end. I watched Emily pull at hers without success, and then pull a little harder; then I watched her face brighten as she realised the problem and lifted the gown before she pulled and it came free. William pulled at his harder and harder. I asked him to think about what he was doing and to try another way, but he just continued to pull. It was such a simple problem to solve and yet it was beyond him. I remember feeling so frustrated and shouting at him about how simple it was, and how stupid he was being – and storming out of the room. I then felt sick at how I'd behaved and was consumed with guilt. As I listened to his tears I realised that I'd just managed to upset my boy and damage his self-esteem in one bad-tempered minute.

When Julie and I argued it would invariably be about how she did too much for William and expected too much from Emily. The reality, though, was it was just self-preservation on her part. William would test the patience of a saint and daily tasks could become massive dramas without her intervention.

There was a Montessori nursey called Old Laburnum that was in a beautiful thatched cottage a few miles from where we lived. It was owned and run by Denise Morrell; she was a fantastic lady and very highly regarded. The twins were enrolled to start there in September 1999, but Emily was ready earlier and so she started around Easter, soon after turning two. Decisions like that were not taken lightly, as we were concerned what the potential impact of separating the twins might be, but we didn't want to slow down Emily's development. Emily thrived there and we were excited at the prospect of what they could do for Will. At the time, it felt to us like everyone else was in denial. There were clearly problems with William's development, but we were still being silenced by the overwhelming majority, who believed it was just a matter of time until he caught up.

We went to our first parents' evening at the Montessori with Denise and, after hearing how well Emily was doing and what a delight she was to have in her class, she moved on to William. She was kind and considerate with her words, but they were still hard to hear. We were told that his concentration was very poor and that he used diversionary tactics to avoid concentrating. He seemed unable to work successfully in a group. He did not talk very much and when he did he used singular words to communicate. If he wanted to play with other children he would just stand in front of them. He could pour his own drink, but couldn't tell when the cup was full. He could not function independently, and appeared to forget what he had been asked to do. He was unable to sit still when asked, and became disruptive. When any task seemed too difficult for him, he would either wander off or fall asleep. So far, he had been unable to complete a single task he'd been set. The only time he was fully engaged was when it was the music session – but then he wanted to be the centre of attention and got upset when he was not. There were a range of emotions we were going through now, and it was clearly upsetting for Julie, but for the first time someone else was telling us we were right: there were clearly issues with William and she was determined to help in any way she could. Finally, we had someone onside to help us get the answers we so badly needed.

Before we had a diagnosis for William there were so many times I questioned our ability as parents and worried we were getting it all wrong. I'd always thought that being a good parent was fundamentally simple: give your children lots of love and teach them right from wrong, and make sure there are clearly defined boundaries, and they will turn out fine. William made me doubt everything in those first few years, and I'm sure if it wasn't for Emily we may have cracked. Our relationship was always strong but in those dark days when Will was pushing us to our limits it was easy to turn on each other and point the blame. I think watching Emily grow up was a constant reminder that we were doing okay, and not to be too hard on ourselves.

Although William had his problems, there was something about him that drew people in; he had a kind of magnetism that I've only seen in a very small number of people. He was a fascinating boy, who was both intriguing and enchanting, but I think the special ingredient was his honesty. Children learn very quickly how to manipulate people and situations to get what they want, but William had no concept of that, he was just pure innocence and acted out his life with no inhibitions. He would open his arms up to cuddle anyone, and genuinely seemed to gravitate to those who needed one, and if they allowed him in you could see the profound effect it had on them. We all know people whose mere presence can drain your energy, but William was the complete opposite and had a remarkable ability to lift your spirits.

I realise now that part of the reason it took so long to get a diagnosis for William was that he was so engaging. Often children with special needs can seem distant, isolated and emotionally detached. But whenever we did take William to the doctors with our concerns, he would brighten the whole surgery with his smiles and cuddles and he'd remember which drawer the sweets were kept in, and that appeared to ease our GP's mind that all was okay. When we went with a letter in hand from Denise, the principal of the

Montessori, setting out all her observations, we were promised that the wheels would be put in motion. They were. But these wheels moved painfully slowly.

A few months went by before we received a letter inviting us to take Will to the child development centre in Poole. After that first appointment, a follow-up one would be booked, and so on. Julie ended up taking him for an appointment every week for over six months, where they would monitor him through play and make notes. About a year later we received notification that he needed to go into Poole Hospital for a brain scan. When he came home, he had to sleep with a cap on that made him look like Doc from the film *Back to the Future*. Then there was more time awaiting results while further appointments were promised. I have a tremendous love for our NHS, and huge respect for all those who work in it, but when you are concerned for your child's health and welfare it can be a very frustrating system.

I had been working from home buying and selling the odd car now for over a year. It was terrific to be around so much with the children, but it wasn't financially viable. We decided to sell the house, as it had risen in value considerably, and we bought another property a couple of miles up the road. We got top money for ours, and a great deal on the new one; it was very similar to buying and selling cars and I seemed to have a talent for it. Julie started working again as a childminder, and our new home was swiftly turned into Fort Knox with toughened glass, locks on every door, and gates on the stairs. I swear it could take me five minutes to move from room to room, so I decided it was time for me to get out and get a job. This in itself was a terrifying prospect having been my own boss for a considerable time; but I knew I couldn't work indoors all day, so decided a field sales role would be ideal.

I applied for a job with an office supplies company that were listed in *The Times* top 100 companies to work for and was invited for an interview. Unfortunately, the date clashed with the day William was due to have an operation to correct his squint, and Julie couldn't take him due to her work commitments. There was no way I could've expected anyone else to take my three-year-old son in for surgery, and I didn't want to postpone either the operation or my interview. I realised that the operation was at Bournemouth hospital and the interview was to be held just five miles away. With a strong wind behind, and a lot of luck, the timing could just about work. I could watch Will go under the anaesthetic and then make a dash to the interview and be back in time to watch him come around. As plans go it was fraught with potential problems . . . and I'd completely overlooked one major issue.

The day arrived and we set off for the hospital. I'd managed to get out of the house in my finest suit without being covered in dog hair or children's breakfast. The traffic was light, and we had an easy journey, arriving in plenty of time, and even managed to find a parking space quickly. We were informed that his operation would be on time, so while Will played with the toys I had a look through my CV and references. I soon realised that I wasn't taking anything in, so I called Will over and put him on my lap and gave him a hug.

"Not long now, Will. It's exciting, isn't it. The really clever doctors are going to make your eyes better."

"Daddy, Dad, where Enwy? Where Umily? Are we go home after?"

"Yes, Will, we'll go home and see them. Who do you love Will?"

"I love Umily, I love Enwy, I love Mummy, I love Umily, I love . . .Daddy, who dat?"

"Oh, Will, I think that's the nurse, it's time to go," I said, as I stood up with him still in my arms.

I realised then that I was becoming emotional. I'd normally take everything in my stride, but my little boy was being so brave and I was really struggling to hold it together.

When eventually we were in theatre, and all ready to go, I said, "I love you, Will."

He was half propped up with a pillow, and as the nurse administered the anaesthetic and started counting slowly backwards from ten, he opened his arms as wide as he could and said, "I love you dis much," and slumped backwards and was asleep before she reached seven.

As his head hit the pillow I immediately welled up and had to leave the room. I hadn't even considered how I would be feeling and now, forty minutes before a job interview, and I was in a hospital toilet splashing water on my face.

As I made my way across town all I could think of was my little man, and when I arrived I had no idea how I'd got there. I was interviewed by a guy called Mark and all I remember of the interview was the conversation we had afterwards. He believed that you learned more about a person having a chat over a coffee, so after the formal interview he invited me to join him. Mark told me he had a son who was only a year old; I told him I had twins who were nearly four, and we joked about sleep deprivation. I explained where William was and apologised that I wasn't able to stay any longer. He couldn't believe that I'd not only attended the interview but done so well under the circumstances. Despite it going against standard company policy, he offered me the job there and then. I got back in my car and drove back to the hospital and only had ten minutes to wait until William woke up. They had operated on both eyes successfully, and although a little groggy he was fine. Despite the obvious success of the day, if you are ever faced with a similar situation I thoroughly recommend you postpone the interview!

Chapter Three

Digging A Hole With Your Face

In September 2001, aged four-and-a-half, William and Emily started their Reception year in their first school. It was about half a mile from our home and we both walked with them on their first day and said our goodbyes at the gate. Emily was quite short for her age, and had long brown hair and dark eyes that were almost oriental-looking. She was a very pretty girl and looked just like her mum. William didn't look like either of us. He was tall and slim and quite pale, with blue-green eyes, and had a narrow jaw and a prominent forehead and wore glasses. They both looked extremely cute, though, and were very proud of their matching school uniforms, and happily walked away from us across the playground hand in hand.

We'd been very lucky to have friends and family who were willing to help out with the twin's care, either babysitting a night, or entire weekends if we could get away – most notably, two of Julie's best friends, Mel and Lydia, who were around so much helping with the twins it was a standing joke that I had three wives. Consequently, the twins were very sociable children and not at all clingy. Not all the parents at the gate that first morning were so fortunate and there were lots of tears and tantrums. I'm sure having each other made the day less daunting for the twins, but we were never ones to instil worry in them anyway. I've witnessed many parents telling their children that if they are brave at the dentist they'll give them a treat, and seen children picked up the moment a dog comes close. Consequently, they learn to believe dentists and dogs are to be feared. We just weren't like that and brought the children up to be quite fearless, and regardless of Will's limitations, both he and his sister were very confident children.

The hardest thing was trying to establish which child was to blame if they'd been naughty, if something had been broken, or a mess had been made. You needed to be a criminal psychologist to get to the bottom of it! Emily was quickly learning that she could blame Will for everything and, when questioned, he would just admit to it. Whatever they got up to as a pair was apparently always William's doing. Emily could get him to do whatever she wanted and then he'd take the blame if it all went wrong.

One evening I went into Emily's bedroom and everything on top of her pine chest of drawers had been either moved or broken, and trinkets and ornaments were all over the place. It made no sense as it was about five feet high and there was no way she could've reached. I decided to say nothing and wait for the mystery to unfold. I only had to wait until the next day to witness Emily pulling out the lower drawers and instructing Will to climb up like a ladder, opening each drawer as he went. It was seriously impressive, albeit potentially dangerous, and under interrogation it was all Will's idea, of course. It was tough, because obviously Emily's lies should be punished; but William's loyalty to his sister was admirable, and he wouldn't back down, even if we threatened to remove his toys. He loved her very much and every night, after we tucked him in and kissed him goodnight, we'd hear him get out of bed and sneak across the landing to get into Emily's bed.

Unfortunately, William's time at his first school was a very unhappy one, as he hadn't yet been diagnosed and his inability to complete tasks was mistaken for poor behaviour. On a daily basis, we would get either a note in his book or a phone call home and it was really tough to deal with. Even worse was when Julie was waiting at the school gates with the other mums – the head teacher would march him across the school and deliver him to Julie while berating her in front of everyone. Sometimes I would come home from work to find Julie either sobbing into her hands or at the business end of a bottle of wine. I have always been fiercely protective of those I love, and if they've been hurt or upset, God help the perpetrator. Fortunately, I am also rational, and always manage to dismiss the first thoughts of killing them and come up with a more civilised method of dealing with it!

One night, after a particularly bad day, I was reading through Will's school notebook. I could not find a single positive comment from his teacher – not one – and I was angry. I wrote some comment next to hers along the lines of '. . . perhaps she could find it within herself to say at least one good thing'. Julie was really cross with me, as she knew that she'd have to deal with the fallout at the gates. Sure enough, at the end of the next school day, the headteacher marched across the playground to find Julie. She shouted at her about what a terrible thing I'd done, and that if I had anything to say I should've directed it to her and not Will's teacher. Julie was embarrassed and upset and was livid with me for causing trouble. I promised I'd sort it and duly made an appointment to go in and see the headteacher the following day.

I arrived for the appointment five minutes early and she kept me waiting for twenty minutes, with no reason given, and certainly no apology. She was a very short woman and obviously took some pleasure in offering me one of those tiny school chairs while she perched high above me at her desk with all the power.

"Mr Matthews, if you have a problem with one of my teachers then it should be me that you direct your comments towards. I will not have you upsetting my teachers," she said sternly.

She was furious and shaking with anger, so I remained silent just a little longer than she was expecting before I said, very slowly and deliberately, "Yes, you are absolutely right, please accept my apologies. I should have spoken to you and not directed my anger towards Will's teacher. However, we are both guilty of that, aren't we? It was me who wrote the comment and yet you decided to shout at my wife. In future, you can rest assured that if your teacher continues to be so negative I shall come to see you straight away."

She looked completely flustered and had to excuse herself to go and get a glass of water. When she returned she was quite apologetic. I explained all about our concerns with William, and how we were trying to find some answers, and that we would very much appreciate her help in future. From that point on the comments became more positive and Julie was never embarrassed at the gates again.

William continued to fall further behind, though, and he developed a habit of falling asleep whenever he couldn't manage a task, which would inevitably lead to him wetting himself. At least twice a week he'd be sent home in a pair of shorts or tracksuit bottoms from the lost and found box. At bedtime, when we read to the twins, Emily would enjoy following the words with her finger; but William would lose interest the moment it felt like work. It was an incredibly frustrating time for me and I'd be lying if I didn't admit there were many times I thought *why me, why have I got a son like this*?

Normal father and son stuff was just not enjoyable. It didn't matter how many times I showed him how to throw and catch a ball, he just couldn't do it, and kicking a football to and fro was pointless, as he could not coordinate his foot to make contact with the ball. Emily had long since abandoned her stabilisers and would ride around our patio turning tight circles on her bike. William struggled to balance, even with the stabilisers. He would regularly ride straight into the fence as he would get distracted and not look in the direction he was pedalling. I became much more patient in those first few years, but it was infuriating trying to teach him anything; it was painstakingly laborious, like digging a hole with your face. When I did lose my patience, I would feel like shit for hours after.

Although I was doing extremely well in the new job and had already been promoted a couple of times I didn't enjoy it. I found it so easy to smash my targets that I started to sneak home from work earlier and earlier. I had converted my garage at home into a gym, with all of my punch bags and speed balls hung up, and whenever I needed to let off some steam I would be in there smashing the crap out of them. If I wasn't punching bags, then I would go for really long walks with Henry through the woods. Sometimes it was just harder to cope with William, so rather than take it out on him I'd go and clear my head.

One such day, I grabbed Henry's lead and told Julie I was going for a walk and left through the gate in the back garden. The woods were only a few hundred yards away through a housing estate and you could lose yourself there for a couple of hours. I was gone for nearly an hour when Julie called my mobile and said, "Sorry to bother you, darling, I know it's stupid, but you have got William, haven't you?"

"No, what do you mean?" I said, slightly panicked.

"Please tell me you're joking? He followed you out of the gate!" she shouted.

If you've ever lost a child you'll understand that feeling of complete desperation; the panic and fear you experience is like nothing else. Logic and rational thinking go out of the window and you start to imagine the very worst. I was still over a mile away, and I started to sprint as fast as I could while shouting his name continuously. Despite countless conversations with William about strangers, we both knew he would get into anyone's car – and now he'd been missing for an hour. I was terrified and running faster and faster, still screaming his name. Now I could hear Julie shouting as I neared the house. As we approached each other, neighbours were starting to come out of their gardens. They could tell this was real panic, and suddenly we had a small army all calling his name and running around the estate. We searched everywhere, while people tried to reassure us. As hard as I tried to force the images from my mind, all I could visualise was some dirty rotten paedophile driving away with my son. Never in my life had I run so fast for so long. I was fit, but this was pure adrenaline pushing me on. My chest was pounding and I started to feel dizzy and, just as I thought I might pass out, I saw William being led out of a gate by a frail old lady. She was holding his hand and all I could hear was his little voice repeating the same three words over and over, "I am Will, I am Will, I am Will."

I ran over and picked him up and squeezed him close. I could hear Julie sobbing with relief.

That night, when I put him to bed, I stayed by his side for ages and watched him sleep. He was so vulnerable and I knew we had to do something to keep him safe. That was the first time I had the idea that we should live in Chettle – the beautiful village where Julie had grown up. It was an idyllic place, where everyone knew each other, and even the sign as you entered said, 'Please drive slowly, free-range children.' This was the childhood I wanted for the twins, a place where they could play outside all day and be safe, make camps in the woods and build bonfires in the garden. It wouldn't be easy, though, as the entire village was owned by one family and there was a waiting list for cottages to rent. I'd bought my first house when I was twenty and it was difficult to imagine renting – and also having to toe the line. Rents were cheap in Chettle but tenants were expected to muck in and help around the village, and whenever Julie had told me of her upbringing she'd always laughed and said I'd never put up with it. Actually, I loved the community spirit of the village and everyone I'd met who lived there. Painting village halls or running a fete stall certainly wasn't my thing, but I knew now where William would be free to be himself, so it was up to me to make it happen.

A couple of weeks later we were sitting with the head of Paediatrics at Poole Hospital . . . and she told us they had diagnosed William as 47XYY. It was a day of mixed emotions for us, after nearly five years and so many battles. To find out what was wrong was a huge relief, but now our son had a label and life would always be that bit different. I remember being told that it was no one's fault, and these things just happen, but that we should think very carefully about having any more children. The strangest thing about that is we just nodded our heads and, to this day, I have no idea why I didn't question that further. Did she mean because it would happen again? Was it simply because we had enormous challenges ahead? For someone as forthright and confident as me it remains a mystery why I just sat there nodding.

She also told us to be very sceptical about what we read on the internet about the condition. She explained that very little research had been done recently, and anything we read about XYY would have been written over twenty years before. Of course, I completely ignored her and raced home to read everything I could. There have been some brilliant articles written about the condition since, but what I read that day horrified me: boys with XYY will be far more aggressive; many more than would normally be expected will end up in prison; serial killers were claimed to have the extra Y; boys display challenging behaviours, have low intelligence, poor muscle growth, bad acne, and in almost all cases they get very tall. Well thank the Lord for some good news: I always wanted to be six foot three inches, and yet foolishly stopped growing at five feet nine inches. At least I'd have a tall son! It was a lot to take in, but there was an awful lot to be grateful for too. We had been so concerned for such a long time and finally we had an answer. It wasn't life-limiting, he wasn't brain damaged, it wasn't some incurable condition that would continue to get worse . . . and Julie and I weren't related (these things do go through your mind), and surely with good parenting our son wouldn't kill anyone?

There was definitely a change for us as a family when we finally got William's diagnosis. On a practical level, he would now be statemented every year by the education authority; but, for us personally, learning that William was XYY helped enormously. It's always much easier to deal with challenges when you are prepared for them, and it was a massive relief that it wasn't something more serious. I can't imagine what it must be like to live with the knowledge that you will outlive your child, to witness the slow painful cruelty of disease, or to have a child who's either severely physically or mentally handicapped, or covered in terrible sores that need constant bathing and dressing. I genuinely don't know how some parents cope and they have my greatest sympathies. William had developmental delays, learning problems, and needed speech therapy, but it was nothing compared to others, and we felt very fortunate.

I'd read somewhere that if one of our senses is weak then another may be stronger, like a blind person with excellent hearing. I guess I spent a lot of time thinking one day I'd discover William's special gift. Maybe he'd be able to count cards like Dustin Hoffman's character in *Rain Man* and could win a fortune at the casino; perhaps one day he'd just sit down at a piano and play like Mozart. Although it wasn't quite so specific, I truly believed that William's gift had been staring me in the face for many years: his ability to make people laugh, to make people feel better. Could there be a better or more valuable gift than that? William was simply very funny and he wanted nothing more than to make people smile. I had no experience whatsoever of dealing with anyone with special needs, all I knew was my son couldn't be just a label. I wasn't going to allow his condition to define him, and he wasn't just a boy with an extra chromosome, he was William Matthews, who had his own character and personality.

Managing William's behaviour whenever we went out was always challenging, though, as it wasn't like he was just plain naughty or unruly, it was that he simply acted in a way that my life experiences hadn't prepared me for. If I told Emily to get down off the table as it was dangerous she would do so straight away, not because she was obedient, but because she would have picked up on the tone of my voice and sensed the obvious danger. William would always do the exact opposite to what I would expect him to do. The best way I can explain it is like this: I drive cars and have been doing so for nearly thirty years. If I'm a passenger in someone's car, for me to feel safe they need to make the same decisions as I would if I was the driver. If they slow down when I'd have sped up, or overtake when I wouldn't, I start to feel very uncomfortable. Living with William is like being that passenger, along for the ride with absolutely no clue as to what he's going to do next. It's both exciting and exhausting at the same time, and whenever we took him out it was like playing a game of Russian roulette.

One day we were at my mum and dad's and William was having fun chasing their dog Denver around the house – Denver was Henry's son. After a while, my dad became annoyed and so asked him to stop. Will completely ignored him and carried on, so my dad grabbed

Denver's collar and held him close, which ended the game. William was clearly unhappy, and he walked towards my dad and deliberately trod on Denver's foot – it was done gently but obviously as an act of defiance towards his grandfather. My dad went ballistic and shouted so loudly at William I thought he was bound to burst into tears. William left the room, and my mum started arguing with my dad saying he'd gone far too far and that poor William must be terrified. It was a fair point, as my dad was a bloody scary guy, and I reckon the neighbours for a mile around would have heard him! About two minutes later, when everything had calmed down, William walked back into the room, and we all glanced in his direction to see if he was okay. He fixed my dad's eyes, and walked very deliberately towards the couch he was sitting on . . . and picked his foot up high and trod down on my dad's foot. He even left it there for a few seconds more to add insult to the injury. I thought my dad was going to explode, so I adopted the brace position, but he just stared at William, completely dumbfounded. William never said a word and carried on playing with Denver.

We learned over time that William took things very literally, so consequently we had to choose our words very carefully. One day, during one of our missions to get out of the house on time, we were running very late and I was stressed. William was standing in my way daydreaming, as he often did, so I shouted at him, "For God's sake, William, shake a leg!"

You can imagine how shit I felt when I turned around and he was actually shaking his leg, while trying to balance on the other.

On another day, in the height of summer, Julie was at a packed Bournemouth beach with the twins and some friends. William ran up to her saying he needed the toilet, and judging by the way he was holding himself there was no time to reach one – he was obviously desperate so she pulled him in close and whispered, "Just wee in the sea, William, everyone does."

He did exactly that. He walked down to the shoreline and, in front of the entire beach, he pulled his shorts down to his ankles and peed high and proud, creating an impressive six-foot arc. It might not have been so bad but for Emily running towards her mum shouting, "Oh my god, Mummy, William's weeing in the sea!"

During a school holiday, Julie took the twins to Blandford swimming pool. The pool was packed, and they hadn't been in long when, despite earlier insisting that he'd been, William decided that he really needed the toilet. Emily was a strong swimmer and was doing lengths, but Julie couldn't see her, so she pointed to where the gents changing room was and told William that's where you go. She watched him climb out of the pool and run around the edge and, as he entered the correct area, she turned her attention back to spotting Emily. By the time she'd seen Emily and looked back towards William he was standing in the pool of chlorinated water you clean your feet in, shorts at his ankles, peeing up against the side. You can imagine Julie's despair as each lifeguard's whistle seemed to blow at the same time and everyone turned to watch our son's impressive peeing. Will didn't care.

Like all parents, you learn as you go, and over time we realised that routine was vital for William. He always needed much more sleep than Emily and tiredness was almost always the reason behind any bad behaviour. He couldn't tell the time so, for him, if it was light it was time to get up and if it was dark he was tired. Twice a year, when the clocks changed, it would completely throw his body clock off kilter – that's, of course, if we'd remembered!

We went away for a long weekend in Cornwall and were staying in a large static caravan with the twins and our friends, Steve and Emma – they live in a lovely village near Derby and I'd first met them a few years previously on a ferry crossing between Cherbourg and Poole. As we were both on motorbikes at the time, they asked me if I would look after their stuff while they showered. My first impression of Steve was he looked like an American wrestler. He was a really big guy, with a shaved head and a goatee beard, and obviously spent a lot of time in the gym. Emma was a pretty, petite blonde, and she was clearly a very confident and capable woman. When they returned, we got chatting, and just hit it off straight away and are still great friends twenty years later. They are both lawyers and, like us, enjoy a drink – even now, when we really should know better, the quality of the weekend spent together is measured by how many empty bottles of wine there are! This particular weekend in Cornwall was no different, and bleary-eyed we all got up and headed to the beach for a long walk to blow the cobwebs away.

It was the last Sunday of October 2001, and previously we'd spotted a great-looking pub that always looked busy, so the plan was to build up an appetite on a long windy walk and be the first ones in at twelve o'clock for a nice Sunday lunch. We walked several miles, whilst debating who had the worst hangover, and arrived at the pub just as the first few spots of rain fell. The car park was practically empty and so we approached the front door with trepidation, dreading that this was the only pub in Cornwall that didn't open on Sundays. It was open, and we were greeted by the landlady, who had a face that could strip paint.

"Is the pub open, we were hoping to have a Sunday lunch?" I enquired politely.

"You can't order food until twelve o'clock, but you can have a drink," she barked at me.

"Okay, we'll wait the ten minutes, then, if that's okay?" I replied quite sarcastically.

"You'll wait longer than that, love, the clocks went back last night," she replied, and gave me a look that confirmed she was the smart one and I was just another dumb tourist.

We took a table and spent the next hour berating ourselves on our stupidity and how we'd foolishly missed out on an hour's sleep, and Steve and I consoled ourselves while exploring the life-giving properties of a pint of Guinness. As the pub started to fill up, Emma pointed out that the food must be good as all these customers couldn't be coming in for the warm welcome! We managed to keep the twins entertained with some old colouring books and eventually were allowed to order our lunch. When we estimated the food would shortly be arriving, Julie took Emily and I took Will to the toilets. Will just stood there, refusing to go, adamant as ever that he didn't need a wee, so while I went he stood by the door taking in his new surroundings.

"Dad, Daddy, Daddy, Dad, what dat, Daddy?" he asked, while pointing at one of those old red fire alarms that instruct you to break the glass in an emergency.

"You know what it is, William, you have them at school. You must never ever push that glass unless there is a real fire! You do understand, William, don't you? It's very important."

"I know, Dad. Me never do dat. Dad, Daddy, Dad, what dat lady moody for? Daddy, Dad why Steve call you idiot? You not idiot, are you, Daddy?"

Some questions were better left unanswered.

No sooner had we sat back down the food started to arrive – and it certainly looked like Emma's theory was correct. We were starving by now, and just as I was enjoying my third mouthful William stood up and announced that he absolutely did now need the toilet.

"Oh, William, for God's sake, you do this every time. You know where it is, go to the toilet and make sure you wash your hands," Julie said.

William had been gone a few minutes, and just as we discussed that perhaps I should go and check on him, the fire alarm started. Fuck me it was loud! It was deafening! And it took a few seconds for me to register the horrible reality.

"Holy shit, Will's done that, he's broken the glass," I said to Julie while dropping my cutlery and sliding out of my chair. Of course, no one else knew of the conversation a few moments before.

"He wouldn't do that, Rich, he knows not to do that!" shouted Julie over the noise.

At that point, the considerably heavy old oak door swung open and Will stepped through with a look of utter panic on his face, hands over his ears and shouted, "Oh my god, Daddy, I did dat!"

Steve just started laughing and said, "Good luck explaining that to Myra Hindley!"

A quick inspection proved that, sure enough, William's curiosity had got the better of him and he had indeed broken the glass and started the alarm. I took William's hand and walked him to the bar with the eyes of about fifty people on us and told him he had to say sorry for what he'd done. The noise was still horrendous, matched only by the landlady's expression. I picked him up, hoping that the sight of my boy's angelic face might soften her somehow.

"I'm berry, berry sorry, is the fur engine coming now?" he said, without nearly enough regret.

She didn't hold back and gave him a massive telling off, and as I carried him back to the table, still trying to offer my apologies, he wriggled free and ran towards the toilet shouting, "Dad, I still need a wee!"

Chapter Four

Perhaps My Love Had Blinded Me

Now the twins are much older it's easier for me to look back and understand why so many normal, everyday tasks were such a challenge for William. There are so many areas where William improved, and yet some fundamental things he never mastered – time will tell if he ever does. William has never been able to read or write, and he has very little concept of money. Not only can he not tell the time, he has great difficulty in understanding the difference between yesterday or tomorrow, days or weeks, and months or years. Reality and fantasy blur into one magical mystery. Many a time a friend has remarked how wonderful it would be to be William for a day. He certainly is one of the happiest people I know.

I have often tried my best to see the world as William does. Imagine if you are in a very busy train station, and all around is boundless written information – signs, adverts, screens, boards, timetables – and yet all of the words are in a language you couldn't possibly understand. You know they are words, but have no idea what they mean. In your pocket you have money, and you know what it is, but you have no idea at all what it can buy you. You know where you live, but have no way of knowing how to get there. You have no idea what the time is, but you're not tired so you are awake. You're not sure which train goes where. All you know is your name. It sounds terrifying doesn't it, like a really scary nightmare. Of course, for William growing up, he always had someone holding his hand, making the decisions for him; all the people he saw he would assume were lovely; and one of those trains might take him to the moon or Disneyland. He was a very happy boy and I suppose he spent all his life living in the moment. Children approach everything with great wonder but, sadly, as they grow up, so much of that is lost. With William he does understand he can't fly, but if I told him there's a magic button behind his head he hasn't found yet, he'd spend a long time searching.

Although William and Emily enjoyed watching television, their absolute favourite thing to do was to listen to music. When they were in Julie's tummy I used to sing to them all the time – it's a sign of how much Julie loved me that she put up with it! If you put me on a Karaoke I think I can sing about ten songs quite well, about twenty more would be passable, and the rest I would murder. I would also sing them to sleep when they were babies, and music was always playing loudly in the house. I think that my CD collection is pretty good, eclectic and mostly pretty cool – not bad considering I was brought up in a family where my dad thought Russ Abbott's 'Atmosphere' was one of the greatest songs ever written. Both the children would sing to their heart's content and dance around the house pretending to be in a band – none of the words Will sang were correct, but they were both in tune – and Emily would pick out various CDs for them and they would turn the lounge into their make-believe studio. I remember walking in one day and William was unaware that I was there. The radio was playing 'Suspicious Minds' and I watched, amazed, as William mimicked every different instrument as he heard it. He seamlessly changed from the electric guitar to the strings, from the drums to the organ, and the bass to the horn, each time pretending to play and always in perfect time.

Wherever we went if William heard music he was like a moth to a flame, especially if it was live music. You couldn't walk past a busker with Will, he would just go and sit down right in front of them and make a scene if we tried to pull him away. Every year in Wimborne, around the middle of June, there is a folk festival, and approximately thirty thousand people converge on the town for the weekend. The atmosphere is fantastic, all the pubs have live bands playing, and the streets are pedestrianised for the whole weekend with stalls, dancing and processions. William was always in his element, fascinated by the strange outfits people wore, and wanted to be on every dance floor right in front of the bands.

In June 2002, we went to the folk festival with some friends. We were sitting on blankets in the sun and enjoying a few beers whilst listening to one of the bands, and William was in eye-sight, sitting just a few feet from the band, and we were watching him pretend to play along. One of the girls invited him up to join them, and handed him a tambourine. We were both a bit apprehensive, and worried he might disrupt their gig, but for the next three songs he shook and hit that tambourine in perfect time to tunes he'd never heard! The crowd gave him so much support, he had a smile from ear-to-ear, and we were so proud of him. Afterwards the band couldn't praise him enough and kept complimenting him on his perfect timing. It was a magical moment. But, for me, it was one of the first times I realised that people knew William had problems just by looking at him. The crowd and the band were being kind because he was a child, but it was more than that: it was because he was a special child. I guess I hadn't ever accepted that he looked that way. Perhaps my love had blinded me.

It had taken me a long time to convince Julie that I would enjoy living in Chettle. She knew very well how much I loved the place, but she was certain I would struggle with village life. It was also a big decision for Julie to move back, as by now she was twenty-seven, and it didn't seem that long ago she was that eighteen-year-old desperate to move out and into the town. One thing we could both agree on, however, was how great it would be for the twins, but especially for William, so we made the decision and I wrote a letter to Chettle Estate asking to be considered for a cottage. Preference was always given to those families with a strong connection to the village, or anyone employed by the Estate, and fortunately, Julie had grown up there and had started working part-time at the hotel in the village. Julie's dad had lived his entire life in Chettle, and her mum had since she was nineteen. They were also very close to the family who owned the village. We had every chance that we would be offered a cottage but, of course, it depended on one becoming available. People rarely want to move out of Chettle!

A short time after I wrote the letter we were told that Ron and June were planning to move out of Granary Cottage, the four-bedroomed property Julie had grown up in. It was too big for them now, and the Estate were going to convert a barn for Ron and June to live in at the other end of the village, next to where they grew their strawberries. We were offered two possibilities: we could rent Granary Cottage, or the Estate were prepared to extend N° 17, a very small thatched cottage neighbouring Julie's parents new property. Granary Cottage was beautiful, and Julie had such fond memories of growing up in it, but it didn't have its own private garden. N° 17 had a huge garden and wonderful views across the fields and beyond to the woods and, if it were extended, could become an incredible family home. Of course, there was just one small matter that had to be taken into consideration: I'd be living right next door to my mother-in-law! Fortunately, we got on famously, and besides, we knew how fantastic it would be for the twins to live next door to their grandparents. We told the Estate our decision and the wheels were put in motion.

It would take several months for planning permission to be granted, and for the work to be carried out so, in the meantime, we put our house on the market. There were many interested buyers, but no offers, until one day we had an offer from a couple – but they hadn't sold their small two-bedroomed house in Poole. I told them we would accept it in part exchange, and that's what we did. We moved into it, and for six months the twins shared a room again, and Julie had a much longer school run to do twice a day. We didn't enjoy our time there at all. We never felt at home and it was very claustrophobic! Finally, we were given a date that we could move into N° 17, so we put the little house on the market and agreed a sale with a completion date to match up. Of course, nothing goes smoothly, and there were several delays to the work on the cottage, meaning we were going to be homeless for about a month.

I was chatting to my friend Simon, who made his living buying and selling houses, and he very kindly offered me a solution. He owned a bungalow that he couldn't sell, and for a very reasonable amount we could rent it on a weekly basis until our cottage was ready. In principal, it was a fantastic idea; what we hadn't considered was that he had fully refurbished it and everything was brand new and very shiny. The day we moved out of Poole and into this bungalow in Ferndown was stressful to say the least. Not only was it now the fourth time we'd moved in as many years, lots of our stuff was already in storage, more was being kept in friends' garages, and with two young children and a big black hairy Labrador, we were moving into a show house that was still on the market! We spent the first day just trying to kind of hover around the house without touching anything, panicking that every time Henry came in from the garden he might do a massive shake and spray mud everywhere. I was like a doorman, checking kids at the door for muddy feet or hands. We had never felt so displaced, but at least it was only for a month . . . or so we thought.

The very next day I got a call from Simon; he seemed really nervous and his voice was trembling, I believe he apologised six times before he'd even delivered the news, and I just about caught the gist of what he was telling me: he'd previously agreed a sale which had fallen through, but the buyer had already done all her conveyancing and was now in a position to proceed – and wanted to move in by the end of the week. We had just finished unpacking. We had to be out in four days.

Strangely, I wasn't at all concerned with the predicament we were now in, but I wasn't looking forward to the conversation I was about to have with Julie. I could still hear my words promising her that, of course, this really was the last move before Chettle. My mind was already in overdrive trying to come up with a solution when Julie walked into the room with a pained expression on her face.

"Darling, please don't be cross with me, but I'm really not happy here, it's just too difficult with the twins. I've had a cloth in my hand ever since we moved in. Mum says we can go and stay with them for a couple of weeks. I know we've unpacked, but I'll do all the packing. Their place is going to be finished before ours so we can stay on at Granary Cottage, and Di says if we can afford a holiday she'll look after the twins for a week."

I smiled, took her in my arms and stroked her hair. And, as I was telling her I thought it was a great idea, I noticed over her shoulder that William was emptying his yogurt pot onto the carpet.

I smiled and said, "I hope you've still got that cloth, darling."

We moved in with Ron and June at Granary Cottage a couple of days later, at the beginning of August 2002. Although the previous weeks had been testing, to say the least, it felt great to have finally moved into Chettle. When I woke up that first morning, I couldn't wait to get up and take Henry for a walk through the fields and into the woods. I came back through the village, and spoke to all the villagers I saw, before stopping at the shop to buy some free-range eggs and a newspaper. The shop is an old, converted Nissen hut that came from Blandford army camp many years before, and although small, you could live perfectly well if you only shopped there. It's laughable, but I remember thinking if I ate boiled eggs on toast while sitting at a big kitchen table reading the paper, that would surely qualify me as a proper country boy.

Ron was born in Chettle in 1922, so by the time we moved in he had turned eighty. He had met June when he was forty, in 1962, after she moved to the village to work in the dairy. She was only nineteen but they fell in love and got married two years later. Ron was fifty-three when Julie was born! Honest hard work and a much younger wife had kept Ron young, and he still worked, growing all of the vegetables for the village hotel, The Castleman. However, I was still concerned that us all being there would be an enormous upheaval for him, so decided Julie and I should get away.

The children were enrolled and due to start at their new school in September, so Julie and I took my mum up on her kind offer to look after the twins and booked a last-minute holiday. It was a week on the Greek island of Cephalonia, and the bargain price should have set the alarm bells ringing. The coach stopped at various beautiful destinations along the way, before pulling over, seemingly in the middle of nowhere outside a tatty apartment block. I leaned over and whispered to Julie that I felt sorry for whoever had to get off here, before the driver shouted, "Matthews, two people."

We stayed still, hoping we'd not heard him correctly, but then he repeated himself so we had to give in and get off the coach. It was horrible, and after checking in we set off in search of civilisation. The described 'ten minutes to the beach and restaurants' was down a mountain that would've tested the resilience of a Sherpa! When we finally reached a restaurant, I assured Julie that everything would look better after a few litres of wine. I spotted a lady clearing tables and, not speaking a word of Greek, I did that stupid British thing where you speak English but just in a weird accent: "Helloa, canner we sitter here?"

She turned to face me and in broad cockney said, "You can sit where you want, love."

Although it wasn't the best holiday, we made the most of it as we really needed some time to ourselves. We always tried to get away on our own once a year. It was important for us as a couple, and it did the children no harm at all to spend some time with family or friends. So far, the children had been on several holidays around Cornwall and Devon, but only abroad once to Spain. William had struggled with the heat, the food and the time difference, but enjoyed it enough that we planned to take them to as many places as we could afford to. Some of my happiest memories as a child were of family holidays.

We returned relaxed and rejuvenated, and Ron and June only had to put up with us for one more week and then they moved into their new home, Gardeners Cottage. It would be another two months before we finally could move out and into No.17, but it didn't matter to us, as we were in Chettle and felt at home for the first time in nearly a year.

Chapter Five

Aren't We Lucky

Sixpenny Handley is a village about five miles from Chettle on the way towards Salisbury. They have a wonderful first school and the twins started there in September 2002, aged five-and-a-half. We were really happy, as all the young children in Chettle went there and so had Julie and her sister. Ron was also once a pupil, but seventy-five years previously. William and Emily had a bus that picked them up in the village outside the shop, but when poor Ron was a child he had to walk there and back every day. The class sizes were very small – so small that the Reception class and Year 1 were held in the same classroom.

Very quickly it became obvious that William wasn't going to cope with the demands on Year 1 pupils, and Julie and I had long discussions with the headteacher, Mrs Latcham. She was a wonderful woman, and a decision was made to keep him back a year and let him do Reception again. Any decision that involved separating the twins was tough, but we had to try, and at this stage no one knew how Will would progress, but he certainly wasn't able to cope with the new workload. To be fair, it was a real shock for us to find out that Emily was also considered a little behind her peers, even though at her last school she was top of the class. I guess it proved how valuable small class sizes were. The school also felt Emily spent too long worrying about what her brother was doing, which affected her learning. Although he'd be in the same classroom, there was enough separation, and it was expected that Emily would soon catch up, and hopefully Will would be able to grasp what he was being taught second time around.

I spent most of William's childhood believing that one day something would just click for him. No parent wants life to be a struggle for their child, and I always held onto the dream that one day a light would just turn on for Will. Maybe it would be a scientific breakthrough, or a new teaching method that might unlock untapped intelligence, and any articles or television programmes that dealt with these areas always got my full attention. In the last few years there has been a huge shift in attitudes to people with disabilities, physical or mental, and everyone seems to have a much better understanding. When Will was a young boy, people could identify someone with Down's syndrome, for instance. And anyone in a wheelchair was obviously physically handicapped. However, the general population's diagnosis of a boy like William would be 'something's not quite right there'! I was just as guilty, as there was no way I could have identified someone as being autistic, for example.

Although Julie and I would never let William's condition excuse bad manners or behaviours, I did find that generally I was too quick to quietly mention that he had special needs. It could be sharing a conversation with another parent at a park, or bumping into an old friend who hadn't met William. We all give away a lot of information without speaking, and I've always been pretty good at reading people and understanding body language. Most people give off the same look when they are trying to ascertain if someone has problems, and as soon as I saw it I'd feel compelled to explain. It's really only in the last few years I've felt comfortable to just introduce Will by his name, without a quiet explanation.

As the building work on N° 17 neared the end, we were able to go in and start decorating the inside. As tenants, we were responsible for that, and purchasing the carpets and sorting out the garden. All our spare time was spent at the cottage, although we did have a tremendous amount of help from June and Susan. Susan, along with her brothers Patrick and Teddy, owned the village and was June's best friend. They were a formidable pair of ladies and had an energy and a work ethic that put us all to shame. I was still selling office supplies Monday to Friday, but by now had got so 'efficient' that I seemed to be at home more than at work! Julie was working about twenty hours a week at the hotel, so between us we were able to manage our jobs, the children and all of the work at the cottage.

The garden was a monumental effort, as it was huge and more closely resembled woodland than a lawn. Fortunately, Ron and June owned every tool and piece of garden machinery you could wish for and, after several weeks of blood, sweat and tears, we were left with just the lovely old apple trees and the start of a beautiful lawn. The twins loved to help, too, which basically involved no more than throwing twigs onto bonfires. Finally, the builders had finished, and we'd done enough to move out of Granary Cottage and into N° 17 in the middle of November. Although we didn't own the house, in just a matter of days we felt happier and more at home than we'd ever felt in the past.

The first Saturday morning in the cottage Julie and I were shattered, so had planned to have a lie in. In practice, what this meant was getting up when the twins woke up and making them breakfast, putting a film on and then retreating back to bed for any undisturbed rest we could get. No sooner had we got back into bed, however, when someone was knocking on the door and we could hear loads of children talking outside. I muttered something like 'You've got to be kidding me' and grabbed my dressing gown and went downstairs and opened the door.

"Hello, is it okay if Will and Emily come out to play?" about seven little voices said in unison.

I said I wasn't really sure; I meant I wasn't actually sure if they could. Megan and Rebecca were amongst them, and I recognised some of the other children, but I wasn't sure if the twins could just go out without us. I left all the children at the door and went to find Julie, who would, of course, be far better qualified to make such a decision, but she was already dressing the twins.

"This is Chettle, Rich, of course they can go out and play. All the children will stick together, they'll be fine," she said while putting Will's shoes on and passing Emily her coat.

"Make sure you stay to the side of the road, watch the cars in the village," I said and gave them both a kiss.

"Yes, Daddy, I'll hold William's hand," Emily said.

"Are you listening, William? Make sure you stay to the side of the road," I repeated.

"No I will," shouted William, as he ran out of the door.

William always got that wrong, and it didn't matter how many times we corrected him and explained it was either yes I will, or no I won't, he continued to say it his way. All children get their words wrong at times, and sometimes their versions can stick. Whenever Emily was looking forward to something, instead of saying she was excited she would always say she was really 'upcited'. We stopped correcting her, as not only was it sweet, to our mind upcited was so much better.

We got back into bed and didn't see or hear from the children again for hours, until all nine of them arrived back at ours with dirty hands and muddy knees. Julie gave them all sandwiches and a drink and then off they went again to finish building a camp. It reminded me so much of my own childhood – and one that just wouldn't have been possible for William in town.

After a couple of months in Chettle, Henry and I had already discovered all the best walks and explored every corner of the woods, which were just shy of one hundred acres. The woods are predominantly beech trees, with some ash and very large old oaks. In early spring, the floor is a carpet of wild garlic, which then gives way to bluebells. It is a spectacular place, full of wildlife, and one of my favourite places to be. Whenever I took the children I made a point of stopping at the top of Home Field and, looking down the hill to our cottage, I would say, 'Aren't we lucky.' This was what my mum said every time she took my brothers, sister and I to the beach, which was every week in the summer. As we drove towards Sandbanks, the first time you'd catch a glimpse of the sea was as you reached the top of Evening Hill in Lilliput, and the view is incredible. Without fail she would always say, 'Look, children!'; but before she could finish we'd all say, as a chorus, 'We know, Mum, aren't we lucky!' She was right, though, we were extremely lucky to live within fifteen minutes of such a beautiful place. Now twenty-odd years later I was passing on the family motto to William and Emily, making sure they too appreciated how lucky we were.

The community spirit is very strong in Chettle and I was getting to know all of the villagers (the population was around ninety and about twenty of them were children). Without exception, I liked everyone I met, and I knew that wherever Will and Emily were in the village they would have several pairs of eyes looking out for them. The villagers get together for various occasions throughout the year and my first experience of one was the fireworks and bonfire night. Everyone meets outside the village hall at six o'clock and the farmer turns up in his tractor, towing a huge trailer with straw bales for seats. They all climb on, carrying plates of homemade food and plenty of drink. The farmer drives up to the field where a huge bonfire will be roaring, and then the trailer becomes the table for all the food. Children run around with sparklers and the adults share good food and conversation.

Money for the fireworks was collected by donations in the shop, and whilst they were enjoyable they were not much better than the kind you'd set off in your own back garden. I knew then that I had found something I could do for the village. I spoke to Kevin, who had taken on the responsibility for many years, and volunteered to take over, which he was delighted about. My friend Paddy's dad Joe owns a firework company, and they do some really amazing displays around the country at some of the biggest shows. They are also an incredibly kind and generous family. I spoke to Joe and Paddy, and they said they would give us a big display for whatever donations we could get together. For the past fifteen years, I have organised the evening and they fire over two thousand pounds-worth of fireworks for us. And we give them whatever we have managed to collect, usually about five hundred pounds. It's become one of the best nights on the Chettle calendar.

There is very little crime in our area other than the odd theft from a barn or a bit of fly-tipping; but, as with all rural areas, there is the age-old problem of poaching. I was shocked to discover that when the alarms go off it is June and Susan who go out looking for the perpetrators, despite many burly men living in the village. I did say they were formidable women! Well, add 'bloody fearless' to that too. They have chased away men who were carrying shotguns in the middle of the night and smashed the lights of escaping vehicles. I volunteered my help, should it ever be needed, and promised to keep my mobile next to my bed every night. I was a decent boxer and martial artist, and I've taught self-defence, and after years of sorting out trouble in pubs have probably been involved in more fights than there are days in a year. Although it would be extremely rare for a situation to turn violent, there was always the possibility and I'd never forgive myself if I wasn't there to help. This was definitely something I could do for the village. I didn't have long to wait.

It was a Saturday night in December, and we'd been to a local pub celebrating somebody's birthday and had just been dropped back home – we'd had a lot to drink. The twins were staying at a friend's house for the night, and Ron and June had gone away for the weekend to visit family. I was having fun trying to balance on one foot while removing a shoe when suddenly there were two loud knocks on the door, it burst open, and in rushed Susan.

"Bloody poachers, Richard, up in the top fields, come on," she shouted in her cut-glass accent and threw me the keys to the truck, already halfway out of the door.

"Susan, I'm pissed, I can't drive," I shouted at her as she turned the corner out of my garden.

"We're not going on the fucking roads, are we, hurry up or we'll lose them!" she screamed.

"Don't punch anyone!" shouted Julie as I flew out of the door.

Within two minutes I was doing fifty miles an hour, bouncing across the fields in a pick-up truck in the pitch-black, with Susan shouting directions to me and pointing towards the lights of the poachers' vehicles. She seemed to be enjoying herself far too much.

"Brilliant job, Richard, that's it, wonderful, fast as you can. We'll get the bastards," she shouted over the noise of the engine.

It was only then that I glanced down and noticed Susan gripping hold of a wooden bannister. It was very sobering. I'm driving as fast as I can towards an unknown number of guys, who were most likely carrying shotguns and probably not wired up right. I'm shit-faced, unarmed, and going into battle with a sixty-seven-year-old woman clutching part of her staircase as a weapon. I've never backed down from any fight, but I can't tell you how relieved I was that they got away.

Chapter Six

On The Merry-Go-Round We Would Go

Despite being held back a year, William continued to struggle with the work at school. Fortunately, the teachers loved him and his personality won them over on many an occasion when his behaviour disrupted the class. He was such a happy boy usually, but we'd noticed some worrying changes in him. He was often in a terrible mood in the mornings, he had started getting nightmares, and he was regularly complaining about tummy aches. It's very common for children to feign illness if they are worried about going to school, but William had no ability to lie. He wasn't pretending to have a tummy ache, he just couldn't explain the feeling he had which was most likely nerves. He would tell us that his tummy was bubbling, or that he had worries in his tummy, which was heart-breaking. It must've been so frustrating for him to be challenged daily with tasks he had no earthly way of completing.

As his behaviour at school became more and more disruptive, in the back of my mind I had all those distressing things I had read about XYY boys. I started to worry that perhaps this was the start of those problems; maybe he was starting to exhibit the first signs of anger and aggression. It was possible, but I refused to believe it. He had already shown in his short life incredible empathy, compassion and kindness to others, but I was really worried that his frustrations might manifest into something far worse.

William was receiving one-to-one teaching a few hours a day, on three days of the week, and it was agreed to try and extend this to every day if the budget would allow. I know this was primarily for Will's education, but the bonus for the teachers was while his attention was occupied by one person he wouldn't be disrupting the class. They had tried everything, like excluding him from lessons when he refused to do his work, or making him miss out on playtime; but the problem was, each time William was asked to leave the room and sit on his own outside of the classroom he was happy. In his mind, he had won, as he didn't have to do the work and he was always content in his own company.

One particularly bad day his teacher was trying a new punishment of making him stay in the classroom while the other children, who had completed their work, chose a toy to play with. William decided to protest by removing an item of clothing and took off a shoe and threw it to one side. The teacher ignored him and asked the class to do the same. He then removed the other shoe, and made a point of announcing that he was going to remove all of his clothes. She still ignored him. Then he took off his socks, one at a time, followed by his jumper, and finally his polo shirt, pausing between each item to check his actions were having the desired effect. She couldn't ignore him anymore as he was obviously in no mood to quit, and she was certain he was fully prepared to get naked in front of the class. He was removed from the classroom – and had won again. With each bad day came more phone calls home, or notes in his diary. At least at this school they were sympathetic to our situation, but it was still incredibly difficult to deal with. As his teacher remarked one day, 'He's not quite six years old, but already he's beating the system.' They were running out of ideas.

As the months went by, Emily caught up with her classmates and she was really happy at Sixpenny Handley; but William was continuing to fall further and further behind. There seemed to be no progress whatsoever, and every week he would come home with numerous educational aids that we would use to try to help him learn. Julie was incredible with him. She was so patient, and would sit for ages trying to get him to interact and learn new skills. She had limitless amounts of patience for that kind of thing. We soon realised that one of William's biggest barriers to learning was his inability to remember three consecutive items. Our conversations with him would go like this:

"William, I want you to say the three words that I say . . . red, blue, yellow."

"Wed-lellow."

"Okay, good try, but you missed one. Listen carefully . . . red, BLUE, yellow."

"Blue-lellow."

"Let's try again Will, really concentrate. RED, BLUE, YELLOW."

"Wed-lellow."

It really didn't matter how slowly, or how many times we repeated ourselves, he could not remember three items in a row. It wouldn't make any difference if it was numbers, animals or family names, he could never get it right. Every day that I played this game with him I would promise myself that I wasn't going to give up until he mastered it. I was incredibly determined in most aspects of my life, and through sport had learned to never give up, but throughout his early childhood I never once managed to get a result. After ten minutes, either he was really fed up or I wanted to knock a wall down. There were times I found it so hard to cope. I loved my children so much, but I felt like I was somehow failing my son. It's a dreadful thing to admit, but there were moments I dreaded somebody else making a breakthrough with him. It would have confirmed my biggest fear that I was doing a bad job. So, then I would try even harder, and on the merry-go-round we would go.

If something was too challenging for Will he would generally just give up, but like the rest of us, at times he would lose his temper if things didn't go his way. Because his vocabulary was very limited, and he had such difficulty articulating his words, he had his own collection of insults that he would throw around when he was annoyed. Sometimes it might be the first random thing that came to him like 'You fat finger', 'Oink-oink head' or 'You big balloon'; but when he was really cross his most common insult was 'You boing-boing head!' It was almost impossible to keep a straight face when he screamed that at you. If we sent him to his room to calm down you'd hear him muttering under his breath, 'Bigger-boing, boing-boing head' as he walked away.

When we lived in Wimborne there was hardly ever an evening when Julie and I would be in on our own. We were such sociable people and every night Julie would share the sofa with Mel, Lydia or Sally, and I'd be sitting at the dining room table playing cards or just drinking and talking bollocks with my mates. After we moved twelve miles away to Chettle understandably the number of friends who'd just drop in reduced dramatically, and it took us a while to come to terms with. I was also struggling to get used to what I referred to as 'Chettle-time'. The word would go around the village that as many people as possible would be required to meet at 6:00pm to help erect a marquee. Bearing in mind that my dog could put up a tent faster than me, it wouldn't be something I was looking forward to. However, I'd be there, right on time, and stand around for twenty minutes before the next person would arrive, followed by the remaining lot in dribs and drabs for the next hour. In my head I'd be fucking screaming, but no one else seemed to care. 'It'll be done when it's done' would be the attitude. Just as my son was teaching me to be far more patient, Chettle was doing the same.

Despite me now only working the bare minimum of hours, I was still smashing all of my targets and was frequently in the top ten in the sales force nationwide out of over four hundred people. I had grown the territory in Bournemouth to an extent where three people were needed to manage it, and I was asked if I'd move to work in North Dorset. It was a no-brainer. It was where I now lived, and no one had done a good job there before, so I could only improve it. After two months of solid hard work, the territory was thriving, and once again I got bored when it got too easy. Looking back, I think I was quite depressed; my job didn't excite me and I had very little motivation.

One evening the children were sitting at the table doing some colouring in. Emily stopped what she was doing and put her felt-tip down.

"Daddy, what do you do for a job?" she asked.

"That's a good question, Emily. Well, you see that paper you're drawing on, and the pens and pencils you are using, I sell them," I said, with as much enthusiasm as I could muster.

She paused for a moment, stopped what she was doing, turned her head to look at me and said with a self-assurance that far exceeded her six years, "That's a really rubbish job, Daddy."

I couldn't argue with her. Don't get me wrong, holding down any job that provides for your family is admirable, but I was really bored. I spoke to Julie, who needed no convincing that I was unhappy, and handed in my notice. I had nothing else lined up but was sure, as always, I'd find a way to make a living. The next week I was asked to attend a meeting at the head office in Telford, with the sales director, and a hotel had been paid for me for the night. He told me I could write my own job description, and asked me what he needed to do to convince me to stay. I was pretty sure he couldn't make selling stationery sexy, so I came up with something realistic. I left Telford with a new job role and a pay rise. I would now be working directly for the sales director managing key accounts and doing sales training for staff. The training side of it I loved. I have always enjoyed teaching. But it was only one day a week. It kept me interested for another few months, but soon the boredom returned and this time I couldn't be persuaded to stay, so I left before I became totally depressed. Once again, I would rely on my ability to sell a few cars from home.

Through endless conversations with the school, and meetings with the relevant local authorities, it was decided that William's education could no longer be met by the state system. There were three suitable special educational schools and Julie and I made appointments and visited each of them. We had to consider not only whether the school could meet William's needs, but also the journey time, as although transport would be provided for William, he would not be able to cope with an extra hour on each end of his day. A couple of the schools were about forty-five minutes away, so by the time the bus had picked up the other children it could take well over an hour to get there. The only one that appeared to tick all the boxes was Beaucroft Foundation School in Colehill, Wimborne. We both knew the school really well, and it had a fantastic reputation, so we met the headteacher, Mr McGill, who we warmed to straight away. He was passionate about his school and his pupils, and the teachers we met all shared his enthusiasm. It was up to us now to fight for William to get a place at our first choice, as we were quickly learning nothing is guaranteed when it comes to schools and budgets.

I have to be honest, I found it really hard visiting the different schools and seeing all of the children with their various disabilities and problems. Once in my life, I'd had reason to visit someone in prison, and I didn't feel at all uncomfortable; but in the schools, I was so far out of my comfort zone. I saw many happy, smiling children, but some were severely physically handicapped, whilst others were having tantrums or shouting out strange repetitive noises. Some were being restrained by teachers to protect them from hurting themselves, and others just stared into space. In places, the schools more closely resembled prisons, with all of the security, but had the feel and smell of a hospital.

I found it really upsetting to think my son belonged in schools like these. At first, I just wanted to get out of there as fast as I could. I felt really uncomfortable, and didn't know how to behave around these children. Some would return a smile, but others would turn away quickly or burst into tears. Growing up in Wimborne, in the seventies, my friends and I were generally good children, but political correctness and the like hadn't been invented. If one of the Beaucroft mini-buses went by we thought it was funny to pull faces or shout names at the children . . . of course, I'm ashamed of that now, but we were just showing off and giving in to peer pressure.

After a painfully long wait, William was eventually granted a place at Beaucroft and, as I was coming to terms with the fact William needed to go to a special school, sometimes my mind would wander and I would think it was my punishment for being a horrible little fucker. Truth is, I wasn't nearly as cruel as a lot of the children I grew up with, so if it were true, all of these schools would be overflowing.

Chapter Seven

An Actor With The Wrong Script

Illiam completed his first and only year at Sixpenny Handley First School. The final day of term, before the summer holiday, was a sad one as we knew it would be the last day the twins would ever go to school together. We explained to Emily why her brother would be joining a new school in September, and although she completely understood she was a little apprehensive about the separation. They loved each other so much and she was already like a little mummy to him, constantly checking that he was alright. Although the three-piece-suite in the lounge would sit six people comfortably, Will and Emily would always huddle up next to each other on one single armchair. Whenever they went out around the village, Emily would try as often as she could to keep hold of his hand and she revelled in her grown-up status.

We told William that we had found him a new school where he would be much happier, where he would have friends just like him. We were always honest with him, and whenever he asked me why he's changing schools I would say, "Well, it's because you have some learning problems, Will, that's all. Some things you just find harder."

Will always replied, "I know, Daddy, but not big pwoblems, just little pwoblems."

That first summer in Chettle my younger brother Pete asked me if we wanted to have his trampoline in our garden. Pete and I had both gone to trampoline classes as children, and whilst I was good enough to do some relatively difficult routines involving somersaults, Pete had the real talent. His natural ability was noticed by a family friend, who bought him the trampoline, and for years it was in our pub garden and we spent countless hours playing on it. It was a very sturdy, traditional, rectangular trampoline, with none of the safety netting of the modern-day round versions. William and Emily loved it and, just like us when we were children, they would spend hours on it having fun with all their friends from around the village. Their favourite thing, though, was when I got on with them because if I timed my landings properly, I could propel them both really high up into the air! Emily could just about land on her feet most of the time, but Will would land in a heap every time and they would both collapse in hysterics. If I put all my weight on one end, I could tip it up, then they would have a race climbing up the elastic ropes on each side until they reached the top. William never really understood competition and didn't mind one bit that Emily won every time. His favourite thing was to throw himself from the top, bouncing and rolling down the forty-five-degree slope, seemingly oblivious to the obvious dangers. Somehow, he never hurt himself.

One day I was cooking lunch in the kitchen while the children were playing on the trampoline. Some days they would just sit for ages on it, chatting away, and it seemed like this was one of those times as I couldn't hear any bouncing, but every ten seconds or so they would laugh hysterically. I heard Julie arrive home and open our front gate, and after a minute she appeared at the door and said somewhat exasperated, "Have you seen what they're doing? Are you happy now, darling? Look what they've learnt from you and your daft family!" and beckoned me to follow her outside.

I left the hob and followed her out into the garden, and saw the twins were standing on the trampoline at opposite ends. At Emily's feet was a bucket of my golf balls.

"Umily hit me, hit me Umily!" Will shouted.

Emily then picked up a golf ball and threw it underarm at Will, who didn't flinch and let the ball hit him on the body. They both then laughed hysterically, until Emily could compose herself enough to throw another well-aimed shot.

The blame is entirely my dad's! When we were children, he invented two imaginatively named games that he taught us to play.

One was called 'No Movesies', which basically involved us throwing a frisbee at each other. We would stand in a large circle, or at opposite ends of the garden, and you were not allowed to move or even flinch, regardless of where it was going to hit you. As painful as it was, it was seriously addictive because if you got hit on the nose by a flying frisbee, you couldn't wait to return the pain with interest! Consequently, we all became bloody brilliant with a frisbee, and you'd never live it down if you chickened out from taking a direct hit.

The other game was 'No Looky-Uppy', and this would normally be played on a golf course. If we had to wait for the players in front to finish the hole, to fill the time we would all stand in a tight circle and lean in putting our heads together. Then one of us would throw a golf ball high in the air. You were not allowed to look up, and you'd just have to hope that it would land on someone else's head. Whenever we had family parties, it wouldn't be too long before another silly game was being played and William and Emily always wanted to join in. They were fearless but, of course, we'd always allow them to hit us and deliberately miss them every time.

It was our first summer in Chettle, so for my birthday in July we organised a really big garden party. We invited all our friends and family and everyone from the village. I spared no expense and got a marquee, bouncy castle, disco, barbeque, and enough food and alcohol for a festival. The morning of the party we drove around the village in a large van collecting all the garden furniture that the villagers had lent me. There were at least one hundred and fifty people there, and it was a beautiful sunny day. I had also booked Graeme Jones, a singer I knew who used to play regularly in my brother's pub with his band Don't Untie the Drummer. I had their CD at home, so William knew and loved all of their songs. It was one of my proudest moments when I joined Graeme on the stage we'd built and together we sang my favourite song of his, 'Deutsche Flower', with William strumming on a guitar. He looked every bit the mini rock star, and the crowd went crazy for him. The more attention he got, the more he played to the crowd, shaking his hips and doing big circular swings with his arm. I thought William's face was going to break from smiling so wide. In that moment he was performing at his own Wembley stadium. Later that night, fuelled by alcohol, everyone started jumping from the trampoline over the side walls onto the bouncy castle, another silly game. Only one person broke a bone in their foot, so all things considered that was quite a good result.

One of the difficulties raising William was he never understood when his moment was over, and he found it very difficult to cope with. For example, he didn't have the capacity to understand that he'd done his one song and now we had to hand back to the professional. Almost always after a massive high would be a terrible low, and one of us would have to take him somewhere quiet to try to explain and cheer him up. Julie and I got so good at noticing the impending tantrum that we developed avoidance tactics and would divert his attention to something else immediately. In many ways, to the outside observer, his behaviour looked like that of a spoiled child having a tantrum because daddy had said no. It was tough, as we were adamant we wouldn't allow him to behave like that, but would then have to deal with the embarrassment of reprimanding him in public. At its simplest terms, it was just immaturity; but it was more complicated than that, as his mind just wasn't able to comprehend these types of situations. I often thought he looked like an actor with the wrong script, struggling to understand his part.

William and Emily were not fussy eaters, unlike me when I was a child. My roast dinner used to consist of just meat, potatoes and tomato sauce, but Julie had brilliantly introduced every fruit and vegetable you could imagine into their diets. Ron and June supplied us on a daily basis with homemade bread, fresh vegetables from their ground, and strawberries throughout the summer. Like all children they loved sweet things, and they got their fair share, but William always had an extraordinary reaction to too much sugar. It had to be seen to be believed. Many children get hyperactive after too many sweets, but William more closely resembled Jim Carey's character from the film *The Mask*. He was almost unrecognisable as the same child, and despite several warnings to friends or family they'd always think one glass of Coke wouldn't do him any harm. I could watch him lick a big coloured candy lollipop and start counting backwards from ten; and by the time I reached one, he'd be climbing the walls and jumping off the furniture.

Although William would happily eat anything, mealtimes were really painful. He was probably the slowest eater I've ever known and would chew each mouthful of food until he'd broken it down to its atoms. It could be his favourite meal in front of him, but when he ate it looked like he was trying to eat three Jacob's Cream Crackers without a glass of water. He would turn his food around and around in his mouth like a washing machine going through a slow cycle. We tried all the usual parenting tricks, like bribery, but it always fell on deaf ears. We tried to sit around the table and eat as a family most evenings, but when he took too long we would leave him on his own to finish his food. He seemed happier then, though, as he was under no pressure and could eat as slowly as he wanted.

The hardest times were if we went out to eat in a restaurant. We'd book an early table, as the children were young, but it would inevitably end up as a late night for them. In those days, I had such massive internal battles going on. All I wanted was to be a normal family who could enjoy going out to eat together and would start every such evening full of optimism. Inevitably, after an hour of trying to get Will to speed up, or battling to keep him awake, I would return to thinking *why do I bother*. Julie was always so calm, and would only need to lean over and rest a hand on mine, or mouth 'I love you' across the table, and I'd feel more able to cope.

Although all mealtimes were a challenge, it wasn't as if William didn't eat. If he woke up before us he would eat at least three bananas in the morning, and if he was really hungry we'd find him eating plain slices of bread; but he wouldn't think to spread anything on it, even though his absolute favourite thing was his nanny June's strawberry jam. (We went through a jar of her homemade jam every couple of weeks!) I was just concerned at how skinny he was, and having come from a family of broad, strong men it was hard to accept. He was physically very weak, and his sister could push him around with ease if she wanted to. Consequently, we spent most days trying to get him to eat and build him up – apart from one notable exception.

Julie has always done the majority of the cooking for the children, but I like to cook for us too. For a few days that summer I was doing it all, as Julie had shut her thumb in the car door – the kind of thing that only happens after a really stressful supermarket shop when you're rushing to load bags and the children into the car. This particular day I was in the garden painting the railings – for me to do any DIY was a miracle, but I was nearly finished and didn't want to stop before the job was done – and a couple of times Julie had leaned out of an upstairs window and reminded me of the time, suggesting that the children must be starving. I ignored her and pushed on regardless, deciding that they'd survive and nothing was going to dent my progress.

When eventually I'd finished and cleaned myself up I went in search of the children to ask them what they fancied for tea. Emily was playing in her room, but I couldn't find William anywhere, and he wasn't responding to my calls, so Julie came downstairs to help. We knew he hadn't left the house, but just as we realised Henry was missing too we heard a little voice coming from the dining room. We crept silently towards the door and peered around the corner to listen to what he was saying. William and the dog were hidden behind the chairs under the table, and next to Will was a large packet of dog biscuits. William was grabbing handfuls of them and whispering to Henry, "One for Enwy, and one for Will."

Henry seemed very happy to be playing this game, and we'll never know how many they had both eaten. Fortunately, William still preferred bananas and strawberry jam sandwiches afterwards!

For the last two weeks of that summer holiday, William was a lion. Our friends had given him a fantastic, life-like fancy dress costume that their child had outgrown and William refused to wear anything else. Julie had to wash it while he was asleep so that he could wear it the following day. It was the happiest I'd ever seen him, and he loved walking around the village and making people laugh. Customers driving into the hotel car park were greeted by a small lion doing a funny dance, or he'd sit on the grass outside the village shop waving as each car or tractor went by. It would be the start of a lifelong obsession with dressing-up costumes, and living in Chettle gave him the freedom to roam freely in whatever outfit he fancied that day. Like the old cartoon character Mr Ben, he would choose a costume and live a new fantasy every day.

Chapter Eight

Well That Went Well

Emily considered it most unfair that first school day in September 2003 when she had to walk down the road on her own to catch her bus outside the village shop. For obvious reasons, the school policy at Beaucroft was pupils would get picked up directly from their homes. William stood at our gate holding his school bag, and as the mini-bus reversed slowly down our driveway we had to shout to stop him running out to greet it. He was very excited and, as the door was opened, he went charging up to jump in. On each mini-bus there was the driver and an escort for the children – in our case a lady called Kim. She slowed Will down, and greeted him warmly; but then had to politely refuse his offer of a cuddle and very calmly explain to him the rules of the bus. He got on very happily, and as I told him to be sure he was a good boy, he turned around in his seat, waved, and said, "No I will," which produced a big smile from Kim – and a look of confusion from the driver.

When Will's bus dropped him back at about four o'clock that first day he was fast asleep. Although Beaucroft was only a fifteen-minute drive, with the route they had to take – to pick up and drop off the different children – the journey could take up to forty-five minutes, which was still considerably less than what he would've had to endure at the other two schools. He was in a bad mood when we woke him up and we just about managed to get him to say thank you to Kim and the driver. The escorts on the buses were vital for ensuring the safety of the children, but they would also pass on comments from the teachers to mums and dads on how the child's day had been. Happily, Will's first day had been a successful one.

Each class in the school had about eight to ten pupils, and which class a child joined was based on ability and the severity of their needs and not just their age. They would stay together for three years and each class would have a teacher and a classroom assistant. Although William had some good days in those first few months, generally we were left thinking *what the hell have we done*. The journey time was really taking it out of him, and if he fell asleep before he got to school he would then be in a terrible mood all morning. When he got home he was sullen and refused to discuss his day with us. We also noticed that he was developing some strange habits, and when we questioned Will on them he would say that this boy or that girl did it, as if that justified it. It might be repeating a silly noise over and over, or kicking his feet out for no reason. He was copying the behaviours of others in his class, I guess like all children do to some degree. It was also very apparent how much he was missing Emily, and he kept crying and saying he wanted to go back to his old school. It was heart-breaking for both of us and we were so worried in those early stages.

After a few months, we had to attend a routine appointment at the school to meet Dr Kelshaw, who was the school doctor and was also a paediatrician at Poole Hospital. We sat in a private room with her and William's teacher and discussed Will's complete background, answering all of her questions on his medical history. Between us we managed to answer all of her questions, and thought we'd remembered all of the tests and examinations William had endured in his seven years. The plan was, after our initial chat, that William would be collected from his classroom so the doctor could meet him too.

She finished making notes and put her pen down, and it was then that I remembered another thing William had been tested for. Without pausing to engage my brain I said, far too quickly, "Oh yes, and there was one more thing, at one point, the doctors thought he might even be suffering from . . ." and then I stopped talking, just as I realised what I was about to say.

The doctor, the teacher and Julie just stared at me as my sentence trailed off. I knew what was in my head was completely wrong, and I fought desperately to remember the correct name of the condition. For what seemed like an inordinate amount of time all I could think of was necrophilia. As hard as I tried to drag the correct word from the far reaches of my brain, all I could visualise was somebody shagging a corpse. I started to laugh, and had to pretend I was laughing at my own forgetfulness. Just in time, before they may have all considered me a lunatic, it came to me, and with a huge relief I slumped back in my chair and said, "Narcolepsy."

Julie came to my rescue before I said anything else and explained that William fell asleep a lot but, thankfully, he didn't have it. I didn't want to say another word, but then it got even worse. Julie was asked to go and collect William from his classroom and the doctor continued to ask me questions, but now more in general, regarding his personality. I reluctantly talked, even though my brain had decided to misfire today and I was bound to cock up again. With as much confidence as I could muster, I told the doctor and his teacher that William had no ability to lie and that he always told the truth. The timing was unbelievable as, just as I was finishing my sentence, I could hear Julie approaching the door, and an irate William was shouting, "But, Mummy, Jamie pushed me and Daddy says if dat happens I should smack him in the mouth."

He may not have articulated his words perfectly but there was no doubt what we'd all just heard. Julie was desperately trying to silence him and I was hoping the ground would swallow me up. I honestly can't remember ever telling Will that, but it was perfectly conceivable that I may have inadvertently said it without thinking, passing on the kind of fatherly advice my dad would've proudly given me. William continued to protest when he entered the room, and I managed to fight the urge to give him one of my looks, as they never had the desired effect on him anyway – he would've just asked why I was looking at him like that. He was then lectured on the school rules about having 'kind hands', but the speech was quite obviously for my benefit! Every now and again I'd catch Julie's eye and, unlike William, I knew exactly what she was saying without talking.

I was so relieved when we finally signed out at reception. Hidden by the counter, I pinched Julie's bum and said sarcastically, "Well, that went well."

Julie smiled, leaned over and whispered in my ear, "You're such a fucking idiot."

I had a great childhood growing up above a large pub with two brothers and a sister. Wimborne was just a giant playground to us, and we spent most of our lives outside on BMX bikes and roller skates or playing sport. I was particularly lucky, as our Auntie Chrissy was my godmother and some of my most exciting times were staying with her in London. Chrissy was a dancer, and one of the founder members in the dance group Hot Gossip that Arlene Phillips had formed – they were known the world over. She then became a very successful choreographer, working with some of the biggest stars like Cliff Richard, Billy Ocean, Village People and Sam Fox when she embarked on her music career. Chrissy was responsible for the famous Bucks Fizz choreography in the Eurovision Song Contest, too, where the girls removed their skirts. She was also in the original cast of the West End show, *Starlight Express*. Staying in London with her I got to experience stuff most children could only dream of: I was drinking Bucks Fizz in Pineapple Studios with Bucks Fizz when the news reached them that they had their first number one single; I got to roller skate around the Starlight Express Theatre; watched Hot Gossip rehearse; had tea at Arlene's house, and even spent the day watching Sam Fox shoot her music video. For a fourteen-year-old boy, whose bedroom wall was covered in *The Sun*'s page three posters, it was the stuff of fantasy.

Through Chrissy I met a guy called Roger Westgate – he was a fascinating man, who worked in film and television. I stayed at his huge house in Wimbledon, and he had a steady stream of celebrity friends turning up on a daily basis. He took me to the TV-am studios, where I met all the presenters. And I was even a child model for a day when Burtons first launched their clothing range at The Prince of

Wales Theatre in 1981. I was determined that William and Emily would get to experience some incredible stuff just as I had as a child.

In early January 2004, the *Queen Mary 2* was due to sail on her maiden voyage from Southampton and my brother Pete had been asked to perform on the ship. He is one of life's lucky people who has managed to turn their hobby into their work – he is a comedy juggler and has worked all over the world on cruise ships. Early on in his career he performed for whole summer seasons with stars such as Cannon & Ball, Lily Savage and Joe Pasquale, to name a few. He even appeared on television with Michael Barrymore and on the TV show *You Bet*. He learnt to juggle and ride unicycles when he was young, and by the age of fourteen he had an act that he performed in various pubs and clubs around our area. His hard work paid off, and he was signed by an agent when he was only sixteen. By the time he was offered the gig on the Queen Mary 2, he was a very established performer and in big demand.

Before the inaugural sailing of any new ship they do what is referred to as a 'shake-down cruise', a short sailing where family and friends of the staff get to go to sea on the ship for a couple of days and any teething problems can be sorted out. Pete asked us if we wanted to go, and both William and Emily's schools agreed to let them take a few days off in term-time. I was so happy that my seven-year-old children were going to get to experience the kind of magical stuff I had.

We boarded the ship with my mum and dad, and some close family friends, and were shown to our rooms. We had two adjoining cabins and, as the twins were too young to sleep on their own, we decided Julie would share with Emily and I'd be in with William. Our only concern was trying to keep William awake long enough to watch the entertainment that night. He fell asleep at the table after dinner but, luckily, we were able to wake him up in time for the shows. The twins loved all of them, but particularly Pete's, and I'll never forget the look on their faces as their uncle came onto the stage to huge applause. They were transfixed by his routine, and William squeezed my hand tighter and tighter as Pete balanced precariously on his six-foot unicycle pretending he was unable to ride it. When he received a standing ovation, William and Emily stood up on their chairs screaming his name and clapping as hard as they could.

As it was then past ten o'clock, Julie kindly offered to take the twins to bed so that I could have a few drinks with my family, the agreement being I'd collect Will from her cabin when I was done. Of course, a few drinks turned into a lot, and I wasn't exactly quiet when I let myself into her cabin and lifted a sleeping Will up and stumbled across the corridor to mine. I put him into bed, and as my head hit the pillow I was fast asleep. The next thing I knew Julie was waking me up at four in the morning and putting William back into bed. He had just been returned to her by another bleary-eyed passenger who'd been woken by William knocking on his door. William had got up and left our cabin to find his mum, and not understanding numbers every cabin door looked the same, he'd knocked on all of them. I wasn't very popular, as you can imagine.

The next day I bravely fought a hellish hangover and did my best to let Julie relax, but William had the devil in him. He was always the same when he hadn't had enough sleep. We were all in or around the swimming pool, and the twins were in the jacuzzi, which they loved, but after a while I had to get them out as a group of about six elderly ladies wanted to get in. William wasn't at all impressed and, unbeknown to me, he silently crept around all of our drinks and removed all the lemon slices. He then hid behind a giant plant and, one by one, threw each slice of lemon into the now full jacuzzi. Within seconds the lemons were creating havoc with the jets, and William appeared from behind the plant, head in his hands and a look of utter panic on his face, and shouted his all-too-familiar phrase, "Oh my god, Daddy, I did dat!"

The ladies all got out, reported my son, and the jacuzzi was shut down for cleaning, which seemed a little excessive. William said he thought the lemons were good for their skin!

In June, later that year, we went to Italy to watch our friends get married and enjoy a week in the sun. When my parents were young and running a pub in London they had an Italian chef called Rinaldo and a cockney waitress called Jan. The two fell in love, married, and became lifelong friends of my mum and dad. They had two daughters, Lisa and Tania, who were very similar ages to me and we got on famously too. Lisa was getting married to a great guy called Richard, and we were all invited to their wedding. Not all my family were able to attend, but as well as the four of us, there was my brother Steve and his two daughters Eleanor and Olivia, my sister Sally, her husband Drex and their son Jamie – Sally was pregnant with their second son Charlie. The wedding was the best I've ever been to, and if you ever get the chance to go to an Italian wedding I highly recommend it! They really know how to celebrate!

We had a fantastic holiday and stayed in a hotel directly overlooking a beautiful beach that stretched for miles in both directions. The sea was only a couple of feet deep for the first hundred yards, so was really safe for the children. Every day Steve, Drex and I kept the packed beach amused with games of No Movesies. One day, Steve said he was going to take his girls out to sea in the dinghy and, if we wanted, he'd take William too so we could close our eyes for an hour. We were really grateful, but that didn't stop me giving Steve the third degree about how careful he had to be with William, as unfortunately, even with family and close friends, nobody ever quite understood how unpredictable William could be. Steve was Will's godfather and he loved him to bits, and we watched Will grab Steve's hand as the four of them walked down the beach and into the sea. Emily was happily building sand castles with Jamie, next to us, so we closed our eyes for some blissful relaxed sunbathing. About an hour later Steve returned with his girls . . . and no sign of William.

"Alright, bruv, fancy a drink?" Steve said.

"Yeah, love one, where's William?" I asked, a little concerned.

"He changed his mind when we got to the sea, so I sent him back to you," Steve said in a relaxed manner.

It then became clear, during a fraught exchange of words, that William had not returned to us at all and he'd now been missing on a foreign beach for at least an hour. Just like the first time we lost him, desperation and panic flooded my mind. I love my brother, but emotions were running really high and it took all of my control not to completely lose it with him. We all started to run up and down the beach calling his name and then, as panic started to take hold, I started running through the surf petrified I'd find our boy floating face down in the sea. This was worse than the time he got lost before, because we were abroad, hardly anyone else spoke English, and Will could barely swim. Everywhere we turned we saw little boys who might be William, but after twenty minutes we still hadn't found him.

As the horror was unfolding in my mind, something told me to stop panicking, to try and think like William. Where would he go? In the far distance, I could hear the faint sound of music and I ran as fast as I could towards it, having to constantly jump from side to side to avoid all of the sunbathers. I frantically scanned the beach as I ran, spotting potential Williams and dismissing them in a split second whilst still screaming his name. People shouted at me as I ran past their towels, kicking sand up, I was sweating profusely, my chest was pounding, and I had that strange metallic taste of adrenaline in my mouth. About three hundred yards down the beach the music became much louder and I spun around and looked away from the sea towards the promenade. Sitting under the wall was a group of heavily tanned Italian teenage boys, spread about on several towels, playing some Euro-pop trash far too loudly through a stereo. Standing next to them was a tall, pale, skinny seven-year-old wearing a floppy hat and a smile, swaying in perfect time to the music.

Chapter Nine

What Kind Of Father?

Most evenings before the children would have their tea they wanted to have a 'bundle' with me, our name for a play fight. Apart from being fantastic fun it was a great way to teach them self-control. If it was dry we might use the trampoline, but more often the lounge was turned into our own wrestling ring. The coffee table was pushed in front of the TV and sofas were pushed back to make enough room. I would then be the master of ceremonies announcing them into the ring.

They would laugh as I invented new names for them and, pretending to have a microphone, I'd say things like, "Please welcome to the ring the master of disaster, the good-looking, hard-hitting, quick-kicking wonder boy, the Chettle kid, William Dudley Matthews!" and he would parade around the lounge with his arms in the air, bowing to the imaginary crowd. "And next, needing no introduction, it's the cyclone of speed, the fists of fury, the powerhouse, the one the only, pretty girl Emily Kay Matthews!" And like Will, Emily would raise her arms up to accept the crowd's adulation.

Then, as they stood side by side ready to unleash hell on me, I'd become the referee.

"Okay, you both know the rules, I want a good clean fight. No biting, no scratching, no pulling hair. Watch the rabbit punches and no throwing me through the windows."

I'd make a ding-ding sound and we'd circle each other threatening the impending pain we were about to inflict on each other.

"I'm gonna smash you into little pieces," Emily would snarl.

"I'm smash pieces," William would try to repeat.

"I'm gonna tear you apart, limb from limb, you're gonna wish you'd never been born," I'd growl back.

Then they'd both launch into me with their little fists flailing and feet kicking. I would block and move, and then throw them onto the sofas pretending I was going to do a Big Daddy splash, but always give them just enough time to escape. Our fights would go on until Julie was shouting that tea would be ready in five minutes, and then I would make them both submit; I would allow them to get the better of me for the duration of the bundle, but I always won in the end. The one and only time I pretended to have lost Emily was really disappointed. She had inherited my competitiveness and never wanted to be gifted a win. She had all the attributes to become a very decent fighter, whether that was in martial arts or boxing if she wanted to. She had excellent coordination, and an almost unnatural strength for a young girl. It was great to know I was bringing up a daughter who would be able to take care of herself, but it was upsetting to accept William's obvious limitations. He wasn't in the least bit competitive, was physically a lot weaker than his sister, and his coordination was so poor he'd spend most of the bundle just falling over.

Although I had long since given up boxing competitively, I always kept my hand in, and whenever I trained William loved to watch me punching the heavy bags and speed balls. I got some small boxing gloves for him and thought it would be a great way to help him to count better and improve his coordination. I would hold the pads and instruct him to throw his left jab, then a straight right, then two left jabs followed by a right hook, and so on. Constantly trying to reinforce his knowledge of left and right and then by adding more combinations he'd be counting without thinking about it. The idea was sound, and now and again he would really concentrate and successfully throw a five-punch combination. It was a tremendous achievement for him to remember in the correct order two left jabs, one right hook, one left uppercut and then a straight right.

When you learn a new skill, it becomes something you can do. But not for William. He would forget very quickly, and the next time we would be back at the very beginning. I'd ask him to repeat what he'd just done and he would throw his right hand first, or he'd only throw three punches. Then he would seemingly forget altogether his left from his right – and the moment he got it wrong he wanted to give up. It was so frustrating, and I did my best to hide that and keep encouraging him, but whatever progress he'd make one day was forgotten the next.

A week or so before the end of his first year at Beaucroft was the annual sports day. It was a beautiful sunny July day and I'd been looking forward to it for weeks. I was fully aware that sports days had changed over the years, and far more emphasis was now placed on the taking part, but I thought for once, amongst these children, William would be able to shine. When I went to Allenbourn Middle School, the year was split into four sports teams, each named after local rivers. I was the captain of the Allen team, but the Stour were the outright favourites to win the sports day. For a young boy, I had great leadership skills and I motivated my team as best I could, and we went on to win. I collected the trophy and raised it above my head in front of the whole school, my mum and dad, and all of the other parents. It was a tremendous feeling and it had a profound effect on me, reinforcing a very strong desire to always win. I thought that if Will could win just one race it would make such a huge difference to him.

When I walked through the school gates and out onto the sports field the difference between what I remembered of my sports days and this were painfully obvious. For a split second, I felt awful that I'd even imagined my son beating the other children as some of them were severely handicapped. Then I noticed another dad giving his son a pep-talk about getting a fast start and I felt better again; I wasn't the only competitive parent there and it was okay to want William to win. I found his class in the corner of the field and went up to say hello. William was so excited when he saw me and wanted to show me off to all his classmates, but the teacher calmed him down and sat them all in a circle and explained what the order of the day would be. I moved back to the painted white side lines and exchanged pleasantries with the other parents.

The first race involved balancing a small bean bag on their heads and running to the finish line, about fifty metres away. When the whistle was blown to start the race, a couple of his classmates ran off while holding the bean bag in place, a few others made some progress but dropped the bag every few steps. William never got off the start line. He just stood there putting it on his head and then watching it fall and picking it up and watching it fall. He just couldn't balance it for any time at all. What made it worse was he kept looking at me and after his fifth attempt he said, "I'm sowry, Daddy," and started crying.

It was bloody heart-breaking and I picked him up to cuddle him and reassure him that he'd tried his best, and that was all that mattered, but he was sobbing and saying sorry over and over. I was really struggling to find the right words to comfort him. I felt dreadful that it was so important to him to impress me, and embarrassed in front of the other mums and dads. I imagined them thinking *what kind of father puts that much pressure on a child such as William*?

He refused to try the egg and spoon race, despite my best efforts to reassure him; but I was eventually able to convince him to have a go at the sack race. When the whistle went he made a couple of tremendous leaps forward, and for a very short time he was leading and the other parents joined in and gave him encouragement, but he then fell over and landed quite heavily and burst into tears again. I made sure he was alright, and waited until he'd stopped crying, and then I told his teacher that I was going to leave. I felt sure my presence was making things worse. I got into my car and drove about half a mile up the road, before pulling over and sobbing my heart out. It was so out of character, but I couldn't stop. It was like the floodgates had opened and all of my emotions just poured out. Frustrations, despair, guilt, anger . . . and an overwhelming feeling that it was all just so unfair. I cried for several minutes and just couldn't seem to pull myself together.

For the first time, I realised that not only did my son belong at this school but he was going to struggle to keep up with his classmates. In the distance, I noticed what I thought was a white transit van driving towards me, so I tried to dry my eyes. As it got closer, I realised it was a Beaucroft mini-bus on the way back to school. As it passed my car I looked out of my window and locked eyes with a girl I'd seen before at the school. She was probably about twelve years old and had Down's syndrome and, as our eyes met, she smiled the most beautiful smile. It was a fleeting moment but I can still see her face now. I sat upright in my seat and looked at my tear-stained face in the mirror and realised I had to stop feeling so damn sorry for myself. With one look that beautiful girl had reminded me that some parents have it so much harder.

I then had an epiphany: I realised I wasn't supposed to be raising two more Richards, but two very different children with their own individual personalities. Even if I hadn't intended to do so, William must have felt an overbearing pressure to try and be like his daddy. I drove home no longer feeling sorry for myself and with a huge weight lifted from my shoulders. I had been carrying a self-imposed responsibility to turn William into a man like me and, for the first time, I realised that wasn't at all what I should be doing. I was supposed to be helping him become the man he wanted to be.

Buying and selling cars from our home in Chettle had proved to be far harder than when we lived in the town. I couldn't keep the cars at home, so I stored them a few miles away, and if I had someone coming to see one I would have to drive over and bring it home. It's also hopeless trying to keep a car clean in Chettle as tractors are up and down the roads all day dropping mud. Everything was stacked against it, and I could go a month without earning a penny, so once again I needed to get myself a proper job. Julie could only work part-time in the hotel because of the twins, and her income was very small, so I had to make sure I provided. I had never found it difficult to get a job, but finding one I enjoyed, that would also allow me to be around to help Julie with the twins, was another story. Within the space of a year I tried everything from selling private health care to phone systems, health products to life insurance, and even cold calling on houses to get them to switch utility companies. With each new job came more training, more time back in a classroom invariably being trained by people I wouldn't have employed.

I went for an interview one day in Basingstoke, for a company that required a team of sales professionals to operate throughout the south. The offices were impressive, but back then I didn't know anyone could rent office space on a daily basis. I was offered a position there and then, and invited to attend a week's training in Cardiff. I had to arrive on a Sunday night and stay until Friday. I hated leaving Julie and the twins, but I set off for Wales on a cold dark November evening and arrived at about eight o'clock. I was expecting a hotel, but the place I was looking at more closely resembled an army barracks due for demolition. I was greeted by a man of about twenty-five wearing a baseball cap and dirty jeans who, despite clearly being English, struggled with the language. He showed me to the accommodation, which looked like a converted village hall. Apparently, I would be sharing it with five others, and he informed me that if I wanted any grub I had to go to the pub. My alarm bells were ringing, so I dared to test his intelligence by asking a few probing questions regarding the company. It transpired it was just starting and they had very little money, hence the accommodation. I think I'd already decided what I was going to do but I asked one final question: "And so, what is it you do for the company?"

"I'm your boss, like, aren't I. Yeah, mate, we'll rock it!" he said, and punched the air.

I put my suitcase back into my car and drove all the way home.

I would start each new job full of enthusiasm, but found it almost impossible to keep my motivation if the work wasn't challenging. Although I was under huge pressure to provide for my family, as the boredom crept in I would feel myself spiralling into something near depression. I would then just give it up, certain in the knowledge that I was no good to Julie or the twins in that state. Somehow, though, I always managed to earn enough to get by and to keep my mental state just the right side of healthy.

I had a friend who had started his own business as an estate agent about the same time I had opened my car showroom. He had progressed from that, and was now running a successful property development company. He started by buying and selling a few run-down houses, and now employed over forty people, building new houses and blocks of flats all over Dorset. Although the main focus of his company was now on new builds, they still purchased properties that required refurbishment. I asked him to help me find a property to buy that I could refurbish and make some money on. I had no mortgage, and just enough money to finance a small project, but at the last minute the deal he'd found for me fell through. He asked me what I was going to do next, and if I'd consider working for him running that side of his business. On the agreement that I would have a free reign to get on with it and be left alone, I took the job and, for the first time in years, I was really happy at work. He told me it would take several months to build relationships with estate agents before I could expect to be offered anything resembling a good buy, and yet, after only four days, I had agreed my first property deal. It's no surprise either that the happier I was during nine to five, the better I was able to deal with the pressures of raising William.

I'm sure in most households up and down the country getting the children ready and out of the house on time for school in the mornings can be stressful. We had a dog to walk, and four of us requiring a shower and breakfast before seven-thirty, so we had to be ruthlessly efficient – and that was never easy with Will. Emily would wake up to her alarm and get straight in the shower, then go to her room and get dressed and come for breakfast when she was called. Of course, she had her bad days, but generally she was very helpful. It was never straightforward with Will. Some days he would walk into our bedroom in the middle of the night confused and half-dressed in his uniform, and most other days we would have to physically remove him from his bed. I'd hear myself saying things like 'Don't you know what time it is?' – and then remember that of course he didn't.

William needed help with every aspect of getting ready. We had to put him in the shower and remind him every day which one was the shampoo and which was the shower gel. Then we had to tell him when it was time to get out, and help him get dressed. Getting him to finish his breakfast on time was a daily challenge, and then he'd need supervision to brush his teeth and hair. We tried our best to do all this in a calm and relaxed manner so that he wasn't upset before school, but it was bloody difficult. There were days when it was obvious William had hardly slept and he'd look like a zombie in the mornings.

One day I was running late and had a meeting to get to. William had been in the shower for over ten minutes and wasn't responding to my calls. Eventually, at the end of my tether, I pulled back the shower curtain . . . and he was just standing there, staring at the wall in a complete daydream, the water missing him and falling to his side.

"William, what on earth are you doing, son? You're not even wet yet!" I screamed in frustration.

He snapped out of his daydream and said, "Sowry, Daddy! Sowry, Dad! What one my hair?" – and picked up the shower gel.

Although he could drive us mad, if he had slept well there was nothing better in the world to wake up to. If he wasn't singing in his room, he'd be in Emily's bed having the funniest random conversations with her. Sometimes we'd wake up to find him standing at the end of our bed just waiting until our eyes opened and then he'd shout, "I'm happy boy today!" and jump up onto our bed for a cuddle.

He may have been a constant challenge but he was also the most loving, kind-hearted boy you could wish for. In any day, he could make you want to scream and shout, and then make you laugh until you cried. He taught me patience and understanding that I didn't think possible, and altered my perspective completely on what was important. The more I learnt to let him be himself, the happier he was becoming.

Chapter Ten

Like A Star From An Old Silent Movie

William's collection of dressing-up costumes was slowly growing and now included Elvis Presley, Mickey Mouse, a clown, the lion and an astronaut. Although he wore them all depending on his mood, his favourite during the summer of 2005 was the astronaut. It was a brilliant-white costume with flashes of silver, a large backpack, and what looked like an upturned fish bowl on his head. Mini-scooters were all the rage, and for most days during the summer holidays Chettle had a small eight-year-old astronaut whizzing around the village. We were pleasantly surprised at how well William balanced on his scooter as he still regularly fell off his bike.

One lovely summer's evening Julie had just started her shift at the hotel. It was just after six o'clock, and there were still a few guests enjoying their last drink after a long lunch party. One gentleman had clearly really enjoyed himself and was slumped in an armchair, staring out of the window, just about managing to hold the remainder of his beer without spilling it. Julie was getting some wine from the bar when she saw a quick flash of white as our little astronaut sped past the window on his scooter heading down through the village. She watched the guy in the armchair do a physical double-take, and then take a long, hard look into his glass, before placing it down on the table and sliding it away to a safe distance. She considered explaining to the inebriated man that he wasn't going mad, but decided it was funnier to leave him questioning his sanity.

No I will

We had really settled well into life in Chettle and by now had got used to the fact that friends would only turn up by invitation and so, almost every weekend, we would have dinner parties. Our friends would inevitably stay over, and Emily would give up her larger bedroom for the night and move into Will's room as he had bunkbeds. Emily came into our room one Sunday morning, looking very concerned after sharing Will's room for the night, and said, "Mummy, Daddy, I don't want to stay in William's room anymore. He was shouting in the night and saying lots of bad words and he was really scaring me."

"What do you mean? What kind of bad words?" asked Julie, while sitting up and taking a sip of tea.

"You know, swear words, bad ones, and I don't want to sleep in his room again."

"Emily, tell me what he was saying, you won't be in trouble for repeating it, just tell us exactly what he said," I said, confident in the knowledge that it couldn't be too bad as I'd never heard him swear before.

"I don't want to say it, it is really naughty, Daddy."

"Well, I want you to, so just tell us what he said, I won't tell you off, I promise." I took a mouthful of my coffee.

"Okay, well, he shouted 'Fuck off, fuck off, I'm not fucking doing it!' He was really shouting it, Dad."

I started to laugh, and quickly put my hand to my mouth to avoid spitting coffee everywhere, but it was now escaping through my nose. I'd never heard Emily swear either, and it just sounded so funny coming from her. I was about to call William in to give him a huge telling off, when Julie pointed out that he was probably having night terrors. We quizzed Emily further, and she agreed that he probably wasn't awake. We managed to make her see the funny side of it, which was just as well as we didn't have a spare room, so she would have to continue to share most weekends. We spoke to William, and he had no recollection of it at all, but he continued to have them once every few weeks from then on. We started warning our friends when they stayed over not to panic if they heard him, and many a funny conversation was shared over breakfast after hearing what new obscenities he'd been screaming in the night.

My Auntie Chrissy and her husband Tony had four boys – Jack, Sam, Harvey and Finnian. Due to the fact that my mum was nine years older than her sister, and Chrissy had waited longer before she had her children, there was a considerable age difference between my cousins and me. Finnian is my godson, and as his mum had been such a fantastic godmother to me I was determined to do as good a job. Finnian was twelve years old the first time he came to stay in Chettle – four years older than the twins. They lived in Bournemouth, so he loved his weekends in the country exploring the woods and shooting air rifles. I loved spending time with Finn and, to be honest, it was great to be able to do stuff like that with him. I could never have let William anywhere near an air rifle as he would've shot his toes off! One day I took Finn, the twins and Henry for a long walk up through the woods, and I was getting increasingly fed up with how much the twins were whinging about stinging nettles. Finnian was just getting on with it, and my so-called country kids were letting me down, so eventually I lost my patience and, with my bare hands, I grabbed a large handful of nettles.

"For heaven's sake, will you stop your moaning? They are stinging nettles, not hurting nettles. You're wearing jeans, anyway! I'm in shorts, look, they don't hurt at all," I shouted as I rubbed them vigorously up and down my legs and arms.

Finnian looked mightily impressed at his godfather's toughness and stared at me with what I thought was admiration – he later admitted it was concern as he thought I'd gone slightly mad. I have to admit it wasn't one of the smartest things I'd ever done, and whilst the odd sting certainly didn't bother me, this felt like I'd taken a swim in a pool of acid. I started to sweat profusely, and as my temperature soared my skin looked like I was mutating into a lizard. Not wanting to lose face, I told them we were now going to play hide-and-seek and I quickly sent them off to hide while I stood behind a tree counting out loud and swearing under my breath.

"ONE, TWO, THREE, FOUR, Jesus Christ on a bike, fuck me that hurts, FIVE, SIX, fuck, fuck, SEVEN, EIGHT, fuck, bollocks, shit, NINE, TEN, coming ready or not!" I shouted and then gave them about another two minutes to hide while I waited for the pain to subside.

Despite being only a few years older Finnian was really good with the twins and showed remarkable patience with William. Finn loved his sleep, and would've happily slept in until at least nine in the morning, but had to put up with Will waking him up at all sorts of ungodly hours. Finn would sleep on the bottom bunk and would regularly be woken by William leaning down from the top bunk saying, "Harbey. Harbey. Harbey. Harbey, are you awake Harbey?

"Go back to sleep, William. And my name is Finnian. Harvey is my brother!"

"Finyan, Finyan, Finyan, Finyan," William would repeat until he was answered.

"What do you want, William?"

"Umm, I like you, Harbey."

It was like Trigger from *Only Fools and Horses,* who always referred to Rodney as Dave. William got it wrong every time, much to our amusement. Sometimes even we got confused with his line of questioning.

"Harbey, you know Finyan? I like Finyan. He is my favourite, but I like you, Harbey."

Poor Finnian. If he wasn't being woken up at the first sign of daylight by a random line of questioning, he was having profanities screamed out loud in the dead of night three feet above him.

The second year at Beaucroft continued much like the first for William. There was some minor progress educationally, but it was so small that it was barely noticeable, the main difference being that he was much happier. And when he'd had a bad night, we'd make sure his escort on the bus would filter that through to his teacher so they could be prepared. His teacher had realised that the one-hour lunch break didn't afford Will enough time to eat all his packed lunch and still get some playtime, so they now allowed him to graze on his food throughout the day. This seemed to be a major breakthrough and it suited William far more. As we were still trying to build him up, his packed lunch looked like Julie was catering for a small wedding, but by the end of the day it was all gone. It was extraordinary how much food he got through in a day, albeit very slowly. His metabolism must've been like a nuclear reactor, as he was still stick-thin.

One of the questions we were routinely asked by friends was what William's future held, and I never truthfully knew how to answer it. To be honest, how many parents know what the future will be like for their children? I couldn't have predicted Emily's back then, and I certainly had no idea what William's would be like. Would he live with us forever? Would he get married? Would he have children himself, or even be able to enjoy a sexual relationship? Would he ever be able to hold down a job? I really didn't know the answers, but I wasn't in the least bit worried. William had such a tremendous character, and even with his limitations I'd have worried more about a person who had very low self-esteem or was truly unhappy.

In July 2006, when the twins were nine years old, we were invited to go on holiday with my boss, his girlfriend and their children to their villa in Marbella. My boss was also called William, and his girlfriend Emma, so it could become a little confusing when calling out for people in the villa. It was an incredible place, situated on a large plot on a mountainside overlooking a golf course, and would've graced any magazine cover. William and Emma had some friends from Bournemouth staying a few miles down the road and they were really keen for us to meet them. Their friends, Les and Julie, had a son called Callum, who was about eighteen and had special needs. Will and Emma felt sure they would be able to give us some great advice based on all their experiences with Callum. We met them one evening at a bar with a large outdoor area, and all the children ran off to play leaving us to chat. I warmed to them immediately. Callum was carrying a portable DVD player and was wearing large headphones and his mum explained that he loved all things Hollywood. She then asked Callum to remove his headphones and say hello.

Just like William, he saw little need to exchange small pleasantries and dived straight into the important questions – "What is your favourite film? Who is your favourite actor? Have you seen *The Godfather*? Do you like *Rocky*?" – and without pausing for my answers started listing his top ten films in order of preference.

I thought he was lovely, and was really enjoying listening to him, but I could sense his dad's embarrassment . . . and I realised that was exactly how I looked at times when I introduced William to new people. His mum then cut him short and told him to introduce himself properly to me and Julie.

He turned around and looked at Julie for the first time. "Hello, Julie, my mum is called Julie. Julie Andrews played the lead role in *The Sound of Music*. Have you seen it?"

"I have Callum, yes. I really liked that film when I was younger," Julie said, and flashed him a lovely smile.

Callum seemed to study her really closely for a few moments before deciding on his next important question. "So, tell me, Julie, have you ever tried muff-diving?"

I laughed so loudly I made the person walking past me spill their drink. His mum and dad went bright red and quickly started to offer their apologies while Julie very calmly said, "No, I haven't, Callum. I'm married to Richard and I love him."

Callum put his headphones back on and continued to watch his film. There was no doubt how awkward Les and Julie looked, so I put my arm around Les and said with a smile, "Well, thanks for that, Les, I'm not at all worried about the future now. But please don't be embarrassed, my son will probably come over in a minute and ask you if you've ever taken it up the arse!"

We all laughed and spent the remainder of the evening sharing stories. Whilst Callum and William were very different, they both had the ability to put us in very embarrassing situations and we all agreed it was far better to laugh about it than cry. For any parent of a child with special needs, a good sense of humour is probably one of the most important qualities you can possess.

Towards the end of 2006, shortly before Christmas, there was a carol service in Chettle Church. I'm not a big churchgoer, and try to limit my visits to weddings, christenings and funerals, but the twins were going to be singing in the choir, and Emily was doing a solo performance on her keyboard. She was having lessons at school and had practised really hard. The church was full, with most of the villagers and their families and friends there. My parents and my sister had come along to support William and Emily, and we all crammed into the pews still wrapped up in our coats and scarves. The choir was made up of just the youngest children from the village, and they all looked very cute and sang so beautifully that you couldn't help but feel in the Christmas spirit. After a few carols had been sung it was Emily's turn to play, and I managed to catch her eye and give her a reassuring smile just as she was taking her seat in front of her keyboard. The choir were all seated behind her, and William had positioned himself so that he could see the entire congregation.

The church fell silent and Emily began to play and, despite her nerves, she was playing beautifully. We'd had numerous conversations with William about being a good boy, but experience told me it might be a challenge too far for him to behave while the attention was on Emily. While his sister played, he stretched his arms out as far as he could, and did a very long silent yawn and let his head slump to the side as if he'd fallen asleep. He stayed like that for a few seconds, and then slowly picked his head up before rolling his eyes and letting his head slump back down again. In front of me, I could see my brother-in-law Roland's shoulders start to move up and down as he fought back the laughter. My mum, who is notorious for always laughing at inappropriate times, moved her hand up to her mouth as quickly as she could to prevent any noise escaping. And I was desperately trying to catch Will's eye, but he was now in full-blown acting mode and, like a star from an old silent movie, he exaggerated every movement, pretending to fall asleep and slumping to the side, then slowly coming around before repeating the process.

As naughty as it was to play up during his sister's performance it was incredibly funny, and his comic timing was so good it was actually painful not to laugh. All around me were people losing their own battles and starting to laugh while Emily bravely played on. When she finished she got a huge round of applause . . . and behind her William took a bow, still trying to steal her moment.

As soon as the service ended Emily came over, and I picked her up in my arms, gave her a kiss, and said, "Emily, you were amazing, that's the best I've ever heard you play."

"Thank you. But, Daddy, people were laughing, was it me or was William doing something?"

"Oh, darling, it wasn't you, you were brilliant. But yes, William was acting silly behind you."

"I thought so, but I don't mind, he has been quite good, hasn't he?"

I couldn't have been prouder of my daughter in that moment. Nobody would've blamed her if she had been really upset, but she loved and understood her brother, and her maturity belied her nine years. It was too easy to forget how tough it must've been for Emily at times.

When we got home I told Emily I wanted to have a chat, and we went up to her bedroom and sat down on her bed. I told her how very proud I was of her, that I knew how hard she had been practising, and that she'd done an amazing job. I told her how very grown up she had been, and that's when she said she wanted to tell me something.

"Dad, I know the truth about Father Christmas," she said. "I know you and Mummy put the presents there, and I've known it for a while, but don't worry, I promise I won't tell William."

I tried the usual stuff about how you have to believe or he won't come, but I could see it was falling on deaf ears. She absolutely knew, and there was no point anymore in trying to pretend. I explained that she also had to keep the secret from all the other young children, but I could see from her face I needn't have bothered. She told me she knew William would believe it for a very long time and she would never ruin it for him.

Raising William had changed and, I'm sure, improved me in so many ways, but at that moment, I felt completely humbled by my nine-year-old little girl. I gave her a big cuddle and as I left her room I said, "Oh, and one more thing, you need to say a big thank you."

"For what?" she asked, somewhat confused.

"All the presents that I bought that you thought were from Father Christmas!"

She laughed and said, "Thank you, Daddy, I love you."

Chapter Eleven

Verbal Diarrhoea

It was a cold, wet and miserable day in February 2007. I needed something to brighten my mood so I thought it was about time I made good on a promise I'd made Julie eleven years earlier. In 1996, just a few months after getting together, I had booked us a holiday to the Maldives, but had cancelled it when Julie fell pregnant. I promised her we would go one day, when we could afford it again, but with the cost of raising twins and the way my work had been over the years it had become a distant dream. I was in between appointments, and had about an hour to kill, so I walked into a travel agency in Wimborne and told them I wanted to go on holiday to the Maldives and I wasn't leaving until it was booked. Too often in the past I'd had the same idea only to be handed some brochures and, by the time I'd got home and worked out the cost, found several thousand reasons not to book!

The agent was really helpful, and forty-five minutes later I walked out with the confirmation in my hand. As Valentine's Day was only a few days away, I decided to wait until then to break the news. It was so difficult to keep it to myself, however, as William was having a bad few days and pushing our patience to the absolute limits and Julie really needed something to look forward to.

I woke up early on Valentine's Day, got out of bed quietly and took Henry for his walk so that I could wake Julie up with a cup of tea. We never usually celebrated the day, so she wouldn't have been expecting anything.

When I returned, I put her tea down and handed her a large envelope and said, "Good morning, darling, happy Valentine's Day," and gave her a kiss.

"What's this? We don't do Valentine's Day. I haven't got you anything," she said, a little embarrassed.

I smiled and said, "I know that, it's for both of us anyway."

She opened it really slowly, whilst giving me a very quizzical look. Inside were the brochure and a note that instructed her to turn to the appropriate page. I had drawn a big circle around the island and written 'We are going here'.

"Is this a joke? Are you kidding? Are we really going to the Maldives?" she asked, her voice starting to crack.

"It's one hundred percent real, darling and we are going for two weeks. We fly on Valentine's Day next year."

Her eyes started to well up, and then she looked at me as if her next question would be one request too far: "What about William and Emily?"

I smiled and said, "Don't worry, they're coming too," and she started to cry.

We called the twins in and told them where we were going and they started jumping up and down on the bed cheering and clapping. I explained to them that we would fly on a big plane first, and then a sea plane would take us to our island. I told them we would be greeted on a jetty by the staff and they would put flowers around our necks and hand us cocktails and we would snorkel everyday with beautiful fish and turtles. Now Emily and Julie were both crying tears of happiness, which William found hard to understand.

"Why you cryning, Mummy? Why you cryning, Emily?" he asked.

"Because we are happy," they both said in unison.

William looked at me, shrugged his shoulders, rolled his eyes, tutted and said, "Women, hey," and walked out of our room shaking his head.

It wouldn't have been fair to keep it from William and only tell Emily, but I wish I had. He had very little concept of time and on a daily basis he would ask us if we were going on the plane today or were we swimming with the fish tomorrow. It didn't matter how many different ways we tried, we couldn't make him understand how long a year was, he just couldn't comprehend it. As we tucked him into bed at night he'd assure us he understood how long it was to wait and then the first thing he'd say in the morning was 'Are we go on holiday today?' I felt sorry for his teachers, who were hearing about snorkelling and sea planes every day as well, and from then on, we did start to keep things back from Will to protect everyone's sanity. If he was going to be doing something exciting at the weekend, we'd tell him on Thursday, and a couple of days seemed to be about right; he could cope with that amount of waiting, and we could cope with two days of constant questioning.

I was chatting with my brother Steve one evening at his flat in Bournemouth. He had by now given up the pub trade and was working as a steel erector, something we'd both done when we were younger. (Steve could turn his hand to anything, whereas I could just about cope with bolting bits of steel together.) I was explaining how every time friends stayed Emily had to move in with William, and the older they got the less practical it was becoming. I told him I was considering buying a log cabin to put at the end of the garden that our friends could sleep in when they stayed, and before I knew it Steve was sketching his own design and costing it out for me.

When I left at the end of the evening I had in my hands a fantastic image of a wooden lodge raised off the ground on a steel frame. It had a lounge and a bedroom, and the windows were strategically placed to make the most of the best views from the end of our garden. The next day I showed it to Julie, and she just smiled and made a comment about it being a 'man cave'. I couldn't deny it. I was already planning in my mind card nights with the boys and parties where we could make as much noise as we wanted. There would be a great sound system, leather sofas, gym equipment, sports memorabilia on the walls, wine racks and a beer fridge. Having a place for our guests to sleep had started out as the driving force, but to my mind was now just a bonus. I called the Estate office, Susan and Teddy gave me permission to have it built, and Steve said he could start around the middle of April.

The last two weeks of April 2007 were beautiful, the sun never stopped shining, and Steve and two of his guys worked tirelessly and finished building by the end of the month. It far exceeded my expectations and by the time I'd furnished it I would have happily moved in. I was struggling to think of an appropriate name for it, when my sister-in-law Rachel suggested The Retreat. What she didn't know was, when I was a young boy, my gran lived in a bungalow at the end of a long gravel track called The Retreat. I had such fond memories of the time I spent there, so it was the perfect name. The first guests to stay the night were my two best friends – Darren was abroad most of the year but happened to be in the country, and Steve came down from Derby the following week – and Emily was thrilled that she no longer had to give up her bedroom. I thought I was just building guest accommodation; I could never have known then that the space we created would make such a remarkable difference, and form such an intrinsic part of our lives over the next ten years.

When friends like Darren and Steve stayed it was always interesting to hear how they thought William had changed and grown up. As months could go by between visits they were best placed to notice the changes, and they both thought that there were vast improvements. Steve thought Will's conversation was improving dramatically, and Darren said he was definitely calmer and less manic. I agreed with both of them. In fact, sometimes Will was easier to deal with than his headstrong sister.

One morning, before school, Emily appeared from her bedroom dressed in her own clothes. I asked her why she wasn't in her uniform and she reminded me that it was Red Nose Day and they could wear what they wanted to school. In the space of the next thirty minutes she must've changed outfits about five times, each time throwing the discarded clothes on the floor and shouting at her mum indiscriminately about items she couldn't find in her drawers. William then appeared from his room half-dressed in his uniform. After checking with Julie that his school had the same policy, I told him he was allowed to wear whatever he wanted that day. He just smiled and returned to his bedroom. Ten minutes later he walked into the kitchen dressed from head to toe as a clown. He was wearing the enormous shoes, bright spotted trousers, a yellow waistcoat, an oversized bowtie, a large blue wig, white gloves and a shiny red nose.

"Is this alwight, Daddy? My teacher won't be cwoss with me?"

I laughed out loud and said, "No, Will, she won't be cross, you look great."

I remember thinking how few ten-year-old boys would go to school dressed like that and not be embarrassed. All he wanted to do was to make people laugh. As he climbed aboard his mini-bus, we shouted goodbye and waved to him, and he turned around without saying a word and just blew a big raspberry at us.

One evening I was supervising William brushing his teeth – he would usually do it on his own and then come downstairs and blow his fresh breath on us to prove he'd done a good job. We'd noticed he was getting a little lazy and he'd started to just shout goodnight and disappear off to his room. I reminded him how the dentist told him to clean them, but when I asked him to pick his tongue up so he could clean behind his bottom teeth he couldn't seem to do it. I called Julie in, and after several minutes of studying the inside of his mouth, we both agreed he was tongue-tied. We couldn't believe it at first and tried every way to get him to lift his tongue. How had we never noticed before? How was it missed when he was a baby and struggling to breastfeed? How had his dentist never mentioned it or, more to the point, his speech therapist? We felt dreadful, and spent the majority of the evening berating ourselves as awful parents and wondering whether we'd just discovered the solution to his speech problems and slow eating.

Julie made an appointment and took him to see our GP, and after a quick inspection he agreed that we were indeed correct. He explained that although it was a very simple procedure for babies, as William was now ten years old he would need to have the operation under general anaesthetic. There was very little risk, and the potential benefits were obvious, so we asked the doctor to book him in. After a couple of months William had the operation and was only allowed to eat soft foods for a couple of days. As with all things with

William, progress was very slow, and there wasn't any kind of overnight difference in Will's speech or eating habits. However, some months later, we were sitting at the dining room table and Julie and I glanced at each other as we both noticed William finish his dinner before Emily, for the first time ever.

Later, when the twins went to bed, Julie asked me if I had noticed how much more he was talking; she said it was like he had verbal diarrhoea. I confessed I hadn't really thought about it, but the next morning I realised exactly what she meant. It was like speech for him was a new fun toy! It was really funny, and exhausting at the same time, as every one of his random questions demanded an answer. You just couldn't shut him up from morning until night! But around seven-thirty every evening it was as if he'd run out of oxygen. One minute he'd be talking at a hundred miles an hour, and the next his eyes would be rolling to the back of his head as he slumped in his armchair. Fortunately for us, he always needed a lot of sleep, so we got some peace and quiet every evening.

He was still every bit as honest and direct with anyone he met, and now, with his new-found love of talking, going out and about with him was presenting us with new problems. Julie was out shopping with him one day and he spotted a lady who was dressed head to toe in black, and clearly considered herself to be a Goth. Julie realised just a little too late that William was fixated on her and, as she tried to distract his attention, he said, "Excuse me. I love your outfit. Are you a witch?"

The lady tried to ignore him, but Will had other ideas and just proceeded to ask the question much more loudly. "Excuse me, I said I love your outfit. Are you a witch?" he shouted.

The lady looked embarrassed, but not nearly as much as Julie was as William continued to shout his question as she pulled him from the shop. He would talk to everyone he saw: if it was someone in a wheelchair, he would just bend down and ask what was wrong with their legs; if he saw someone who was overweight, he would ask them if they had eaten too many chips. He did it in a really compassionate way, though, as if it was the most natural, thoughtful question to ask. We always explained to him that what he'd said was inappropriate, but he never understood that the truth wasn't always the right thing to say.

My mum was on a train coming back from London one evening with William after watching a show in the West End. It was an annual treat for him, as he absolutely loved the theatre and they always had a fantastic time together. A man boarded the train and took a seat directly opposite them, and it only took a quick glance for my mum to realise he clearly had some issues. William immediately struck up a conversation with him and told him all about the show he'd just seen. Worryingly, the man told him he was on the way to Winchester to kidnap his young daughter. William was fascinated by the story, and despite my mum's growing concern he continued to talk to the man.

Luckily, the man got up and went to the toilet, and as soon as he was out of earshot my mum said, "William, I think that man is very strange and I don't want you to talk to him anymore, let's just look at these magazines from now on."

William didn't protest and started to flick through a magazine, but the second the man returned to his seat, Will said, "Excuse me, my nana thinks you are stwange. I don't, but she doesn't want me to talk to you anymore."

My mum didn't know where to look, but fortunately the man got off the train at the very next stop. Although his honesty could cause huge embarrassment, there was something so refreshing about it. We spend our lives trying to say the right thing, choosing our words carefully, and not always saying what we mean in case it upsets somebody. Although there were many times I'd wished William could've filtered what he said, I often found myself thinking how much better our lives would be if we were all a bit more honest with each other. What I couldn't have known then, though, was that our life was about to take a devastating turn, and William's honesty would be relied upon in a very serious incident.

Chapter Twelve

Bad Dream

It was early September 2007, the twins were ten-and-a-half years old and had just started back at school. We'd had a wonderful summer, spending most of the time in the garden. I'd bought a big round swimming pool and the children were in it every day. The garden was full every weekend with friends and family having fun. The Retreat doubled up as pool changing rooms, and those friends that had enjoyed a few too many drinks in the sun stayed over. Life was as good as it gets, work was going well, the children were a delight, and Julie and I were counting down the weeks until we all went on holiday to the Maldives.

I had just viewed a few properties and was heading back to the office in Poole when my mobile rang. It was Julie, and the moment I heard her voice I knew something was terribly wrong. She was fighting back the tears, talking really fast, and making very little sense.

"Rich, something terrible has happened, something really bad, I don't know how to, oh God, at Will's school, he's been, I mean, it's terrible, I don't know how to say it–"

"For heaven's sake calm down, darling, slow down, I can't understand what you're saying."

"It's really bad, Rich, oh my god, please don't do anything, I couldn't bear to lose you, promise me you're not going to do anything stupid," she said, and started crying.

"Julie, darling, I have no idea what you're talking about. Stop crying and tell me what's happened."

She took several big intakes of breath and then said, "William has been attacked, in the showers at school, a sexual attack."

"What the hell do you mean, attacked? By who? Who's told you this? You're not making any sense, Julie, stop talking rubbish! This won't be true, slow down and start again!" I said angrily.

"Please don't go mad! Oh, darling, I'm so scared. At his school, by another boy, the school have just phoned me. The police have been called, oh God, please don't do anything, I can't cope with this," she said, and then started sobbing uncontrollably.

"Darling, listen to me, stop crying. Everything is going to be okay. Breathe, for God's sake, breathe. I promise you I won't do anything stupid. I'm sure it's all just a mistake. I'll go to the school now and phone you after. It'll be okay, I promise," I said reassuringly.

I hung up the phone and immediately called the school and asked to speak to the headteacher. By the speed in which I was put through he was obviously sitting by the phone waiting for my call.

"Hello, Mr Matthews, this is Paul McGill, I've been expecting your call. Has your wife explained to you what has happened?" he said softly.

"She tried to but she wasn't making any sense, please tell me it's not true?" I said sternly.

"We are trying to work out what's happened, it's very difficult as I'm sure you'll understand because of the nature of the children involved, but trust me, Mr Matthews, we are doing all we can. There was an incident in the swimming pool changing rooms and William alleges he was attacked by another boy. I'm sorry to say it was of a sexual nature."

"Alleges! What do you mean alleges? William can't lie! I'm on the way now!" I shouted and hung up.

There were a million feelings running through my mind, each one battling for supremacy, but at that point the anger was winning. I also had an overwhelming feeling of guilt that I'd let my son down because I hadn't been there to protect him. I kept picturing his beautiful, innocent little face and was terrified of how this would change him. I felt sweat running down my back, and my chest felt like it was going to explode. I kept telling myself to stay calm, to think, to rationalise; after all, I didn't know anything yet for sure. I forced myself to breathe slowly. If I couldn't protect Will then, now I had to, I had to be calm. Then my thoughts turned to the boy and, strangely, I felt no anger towards him, he surely didn't know what he was doing. But I wanted to hurt the school, I wanted to pull it apart brick by brick, and I pictured myself knocking the walls down with my fists. How could they have let this happen? Ten minutes after Julie had phoned me I was parking my car and walking through the school gates and a calmness enveloped me. Just like all the times I'd walked into a boxing ring, or approached a group of drunk guys in a pub hell-bent on fighting, I was calm and composed. I took one large final intake of breath, and walked through the door.

Two female members of staff came out to greet me at reception, and for once I wasn't asked to sign in. They kept their heads low, to avoid making eye contact with me, and just ushered me straight through to the headteacher's office. A quick knock and the door was opened for me and I walked in. Seated behind his desk was Mr McGill, with two other male members of staff stood either side of his desk, one of which was the PE teacher. A thought flashed through my mind that there wasn't enough of them, if I was going to lose my temper they should have filled the room.

As Mr McGill stood up and offered me a seat I stared into his eyes – and all I saw was despair. The man looked completely broken, and any anger I had disappeared. He was as white as a sheet, and his voice was shaky.

"Mr Matthews, I can't even imagine how you are feeling. I am so sorry that this has happened. We have let you down, we . . . have let William down. Our children's safety is our number one priority, and something . . . has gone dreadfully wrong. I assure you that we do believe every word that William has said, but obviously, because of the serious nature of the allegation . . . the police will be involved."

As I was listening to him struggle to speak, all thoughts of wanting to hurt the school were gone. This wonderfully brilliant man was so passionate about his school, and he was falling apart in front of me as if his life's work was disappearing through his hands. If it were possible, he looked every bit as hurt by what had happened as I did.

"Please just tell me exactly what happened? Is William okay, is he hurt?" I said.

He composed himself just enough to say, "We don't think William is hurt. It appears that another boy became over-excited in the showers and tried to force himself upon him. William has said that the boy tried to put his penis inside him. Mr Matthews, I am so, so sorry."

For a few seconds his words seemed to just hang in the air, and I suddenly felt really sick.

"Tried or did?" I asked, dreading the answer.

"We believe he tried but wasn't successful. There was another boy present, who raised the alarm, and let's just say that he is quite a reliable witness. However, what William went through would've been extremely traumatic for him, as I'm afraid to say it sounds like there was a lot of aggression involved."

My hands gripped the side of my chair so tightly I felt sure it was going to break.

"Where is my son now? Can you go and get him for me, please?"

"Shall we go and get him together? He's being looked after. I think he's in the staffroom."

"I don't understand how this could've happened, there must be procedures in place to make sure the children are not alone in the showers?" I said as we walked.

"There are, Mr Matthews. It seems we had two female staff on, but no males, so there was no one in with them. It was a terrible mistake and please trust me when I say this will never, ever happen in my school again."

As the staffroom door was opened the first face I saw was William's. He was sitting with a teacher, chatting away, and then he jumped up and ran over and hugged me.

"Dad, do you know what? This boy, right, he tried to put his willy in my bum, and that's very naughty, isn't it? I'm very cwoss with him. Are you cwoss with him as well, Daddy?"

"Yes, Will, I am but that doesn't matter at the moment. All that matters now is that you are alright."

"Can we go in a police car, Daddy? Will that boy go to pwison? I still like him, but he is very naughty, isn't he? I don't have to stay at school now, do I? Can I come home with you now?"

"If that's what you want, Will, of course you can. But we might need to talk to the police. Are you happy to do that?"

"Am I in twouble, Daddy? I told the twuth. Are you not improud of me?"

"I'm very proud of you, and you're not in any trouble at all," I said, and squeezed him tight.

"Listen, Will, Daddy just needs to talk to your headteacher for a little bit and then I'll take you home. I won't be long."

We stepped outside so that we were alone again and, as I offered my hand to him, I said, "I'm going to take Will home now. I know the police will need to talk to him, so give them my number. At the moment, I don't know how I feel about him coming back here, but if he does I don't expect him to ever have to see that boy again."

"You have my word, thank you. I can't imagine how you must be feeling. When you walked into my office I thought you were going to kill me," he said, and made a small nervous laugh.

"So did I," I said, and opened the door and beckoned Will out.

I put Will in the car and put some music on for him, and then walked away out of earshot and phoned Julie. She answered before I heard it ring. I told her everything I'd been told and she completely broke down. She was distraught. She's a really strong girl, but this was too much for her. She kept telling me she couldn't cope and she couldn't stop crying. It felt like a nightmare that you cannot wait to wake up and escape from, but I knew it was a long way from over. As I drove home, William was singing to the songs on the radio, seemingly the same happy boy, without a care or concern in the world. I wasn't sure if it was his coping mechanism or his limited ability to understand the severity of what he'd been through. I turned the radio off and asked him if he wanted to talk about what had happened.

"I didn't want him to do it, Daddy, but he did it anyway. I am very cwoss," he said, matter-of-factly.

"I don't think he understood what he was doing, Will. It was a bad thing, though, and you are a very brave boy. The police will want to ask you questions about what happened, and all you have to do is tell the truth, you are not in any trouble at all. I will always be with you, okay?"

"Yes, okay, Dad," he said, and continued to sing without the radio for back up.

I felt a tiny glimmer of hope: maybe he would be fine; maybe this wasn't going to affect him as we'd imagine it would – and I took strength from Will's attitude. When we got home he ran out of the car and straight into the house, shouting for his mum, and threw his arms around her. He started to tell her what had happened but she stopped him and explained that daddy had told her already and directed him to go and watch some TV. Julie and I moved to the other end of the house and I held her tight while she cried silently into my chest.

I didn't know what would happen next, but I wanted this nightmare to be over as soon as possible. Not understanding the procedure was really frustrating, so I phoned my friend Steve from Derby, who was a criminal lawyer, and explained what had happened. At times like this you find out who your true friends are, and he was absolutely brilliant on the phone. He was compassionate and thoughtful with his words, but also honest enough to tell me straight what I should expect from the next twenty-four hours.

His last words were, "Listen, mate, you're an intelligent guy, and I'm sure you'll have already worked out that this isn't going to end up in court. It's not what you'd want to put Will through, anyway. It's going to be tough on you, but be strong for Julie and Will, and if you need me, I'll come down. I love you, mate."

As I put the phone down I saw a police car pull up outside. I walked out of the house to greet them, but getting out of the car on his own was Adrian, a neighbour of ours from when we lived in Wimborne and a good friend. He was in the police force and was the inspector on duty that day. He told me that he'd seen the incident report come up on screen and immediately got in the car to come and see me. He was a dedicated police officer, but first and foremost a loving father, and he totally understood how I was feeling. William needed to be medically examined as soon as possible, and give a statement, but this required specially trained officers who had the requisite skills to deal with sexual offences involving children. Adrian got on the phone to track them down, and within twenty minutes he had arranged everything for us.

The next twenty-four hours were the hardest of my life. Inside I was falling apart, but I had to stay strong for Will and Julie and get through it as quickly as possible. That night William was medically examined in Dorchester hospital, which was incredibly traumatic to watch, and the following morning he gave his statement to the child protection services. We've all seen images on television of young children using puppets to demonstrate what happened to them, but the sight of my son behind a glass screen describing and reliving his experience was completely devastating.

By late afternoon we were home, and Julie tried to return to some level of normality and started to cook the children's tea and put the hoover round. I grabbed a bottle of wine and told her I needed some time alone in The Retreat, and wandered up the garden. I poured myself a large glass and phoned Steve and recounted the events of the past twenty-four hours, which were pretty much exactly as he'd told me they would be. He offered to get in the car and come down if I needed him, but it was a three-hour drive so I assured him I'd be okay. I thanked him for all his help and tried to say, 'I love you, mate' but my voice cracked, so I hung up quickly, hoping he hadn't heard. My eyes welled up and I spun around and hit the punch bag as hard as I could, and then again and again. I was shouting and screaming, and kept punching it until my lungs felt like they'd burst and my hands were covered in blood. Eventually I collapsed onto the floor with my chest pounding and tried desperately to stop the horrible images that were flooding my mind.

After several minutes laying on the floor I stood up, took a big gulp of wine and walked over to the iPod and put it on shuffle. From a choice of nearly three thousand songs it selected a track called 'Bad Dream' by Ben's Brother. As I listened to the lyrics, my eyes welled up again, and before I knew it I was sobbing uncontrollably. I played that song on repeat for nearly two hours and cried more tears than I had in my lifetime. Eventually Julie opened the door, and when she saw the state of me she threw her arms around me and we stayed like that for ages, two people completely lost in our grief. All she kept saying was she didn't know how I'd been so strong, and told me she loved me over and over.

When we'd finally got ourselves together, we went back down the garden to the cottage and put the children to bed and opened another bottle of wine. Ten minutes later, there was a loud, quick knock on the door – and in walked Steve, exactly three hours after I'd hung up on him.

"Come here, you," he said to Julie, as he grabbed her in his huge arms and she sobbed into his shirt.

I got up and gave him a hug. "How you doing? You okay?" he asked.

"I'm alright, mate, getting there. I can't believe you are here!" I said.

"You'd have done exactly the same for me, mate. Right, where's the fucking wine?"

After a while Julie went to bed, and Steve and I talked into the small hours and demolished several bottles. I told him what an enormous help Adrian had been, and recounted the conversation with the headteacher.

Steve said, "Listen, mate, you're naturally going to feel angry and you've got no one to direct that towards. No doubt if the perpetrator had been an adult I'd have been defending you on a murder charge, but you're going to have to learn to live with this. It's fucking shit, and it won't be easy, but from what you've told me Will's school is bloody amazing. You hand over the duty of care for your son every day to them, and one day it went horribly wrong, but I'm willing to bet it'll be the safest place he could be from now on. Terrible things happen every day and people look for someone to blame, but I reckon those teachers won't have slept any more than you did last night. You and Julie will get through this because you are strong and, because of William's character, he'll be fine."

Steve stayed with us until the following evening, and drove home when the considerable amount of alcohol we'd consumed had left his system. Julie and I took the rest of the week off work to spend time doing nice things with William. We got so much strength from him, as he reverted so quickly to being his beautifully happy and funny, unique self. As expected, the police decided not to take the case further and Adrian called me to explain.

He said, "William gave very good evidence, every word of what he said is believed, and it will be recorded on file that Will was a victim of a crime. I hope you understand, though, it is not in anyone's best interests to take this case any further."

I thanked Adrian for all he'd done for us and told him not to worry, that it was exactly what I was expecting. At the end of the week I called the school and spoke to Mr McGill.

"Mr McGill, I wanted to talk to you and tell you that I don't want you to worry. I could see how badly this has affected you, and I think you and your teachers do an incredible job with the students. One mistake doesn't change that. William is fine, and is excited about coming back to school on Monday."

"Thank you so much, Mr Matthews, I'm so glad to hear that William is okay. As a father, can I ask how you are doing?" he said gently.

"I'm okay, you know, one day at a time. I hope we can put it all behind us now. William loves his school, and we are very grateful for all you do for him."

No I will

I can't pretend I wasn't apprehensive when we sent him off to school on the bus that Monday . . . but no one ever said being a parent was easy.

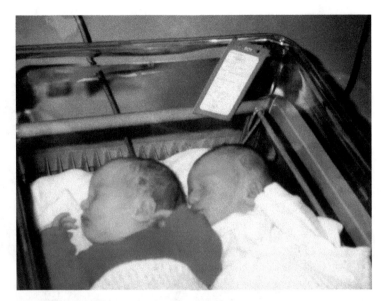

William and Emily, three days old. Will's health improved after I
moved him from his own crib into Emily's.

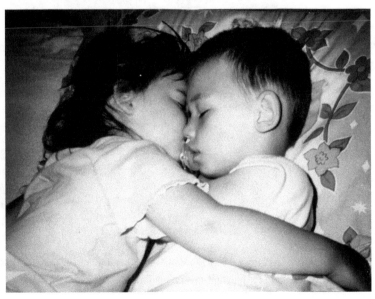

Despite putting them to bed every night in their own beds, we'd
always find them like this in the morning.

no i will

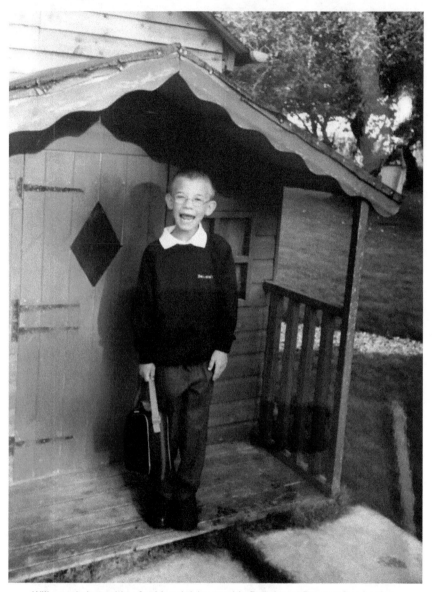

Will, aged six, waiting for his mini-bus on his first day at Beaucroft school.

no i will

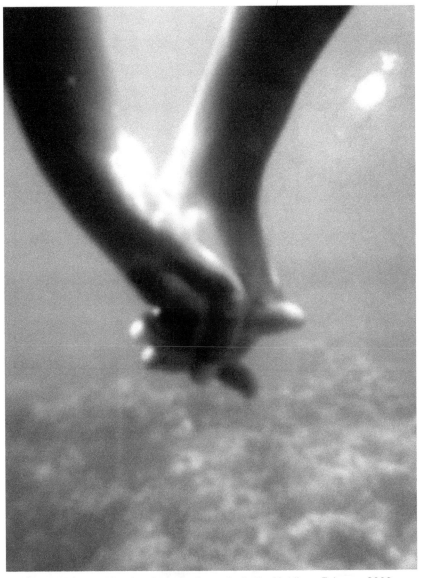

Will and Emily holding hands under the water in the Maldives, February 2008

no I will

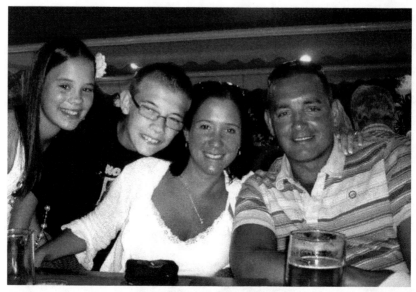

Family holiday in Spain, June 2010

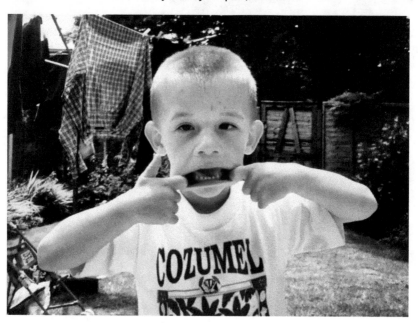

Cheeky little monkey.

no I will

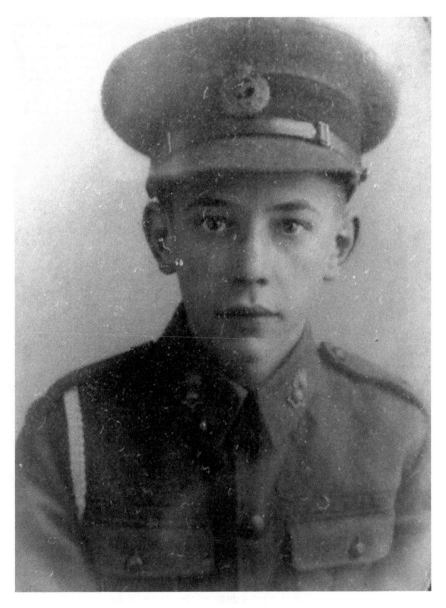

Will's grandad Ron when he joined the army, aged seventeen in 1939.
When I first saw this photo I was convinced it was William.

no i will

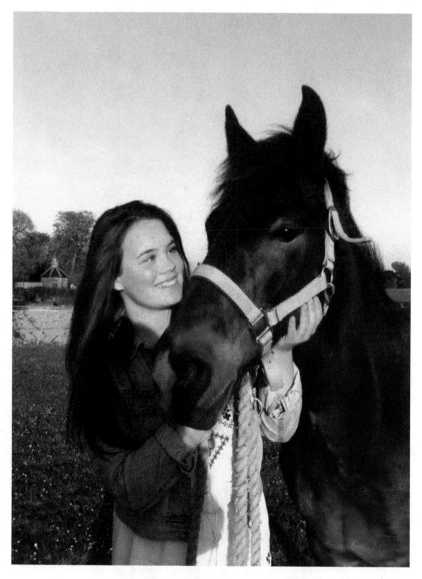

Emily, aged sixteen with her horse Prince.

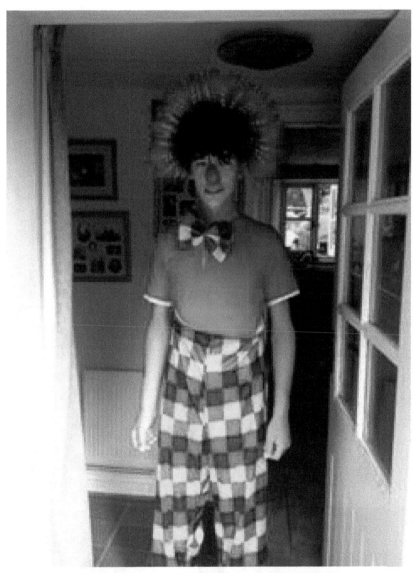

"Is there any reason why you're dressed as a clown?" "Der! I got too hot as Scooby-Doo!"

no i will

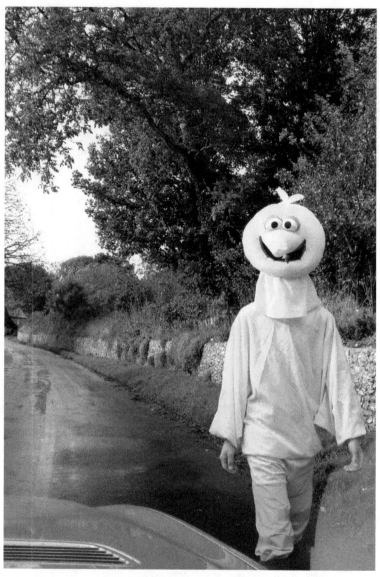

Will dressed as Big Bird just going for a stroll through the village on a Sunday afternoon. As you do.

no i will

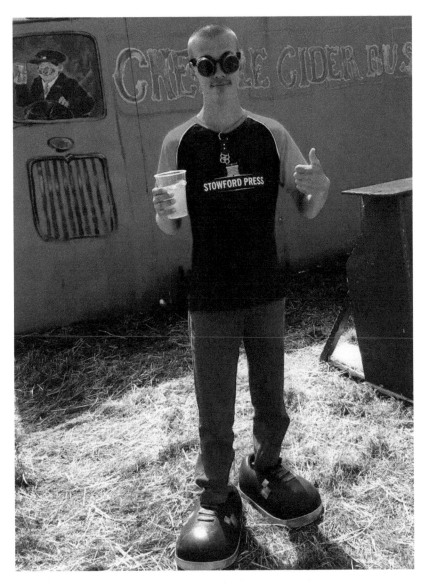

Will aged seventeen at Chettle village fete, July 2014

no i will

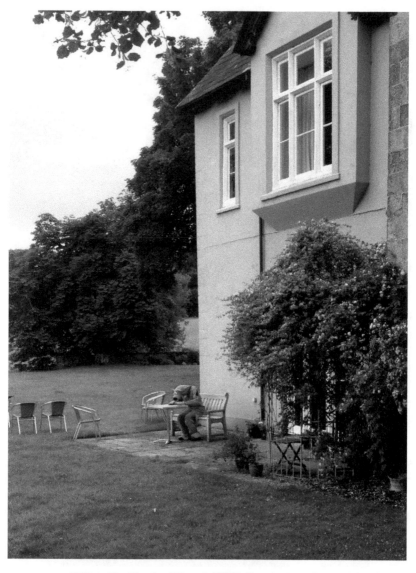

William liked to play 'Where's Will?'. Here he is as Scooby-Doo
outside the Castleman hotel in the village.

no I will

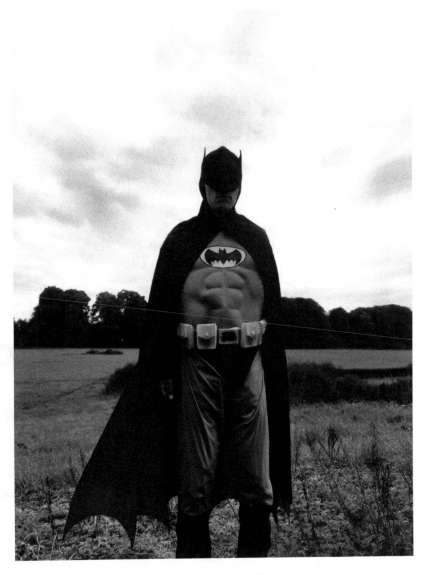

Chettle is crime free when Will is Batman!

no i will

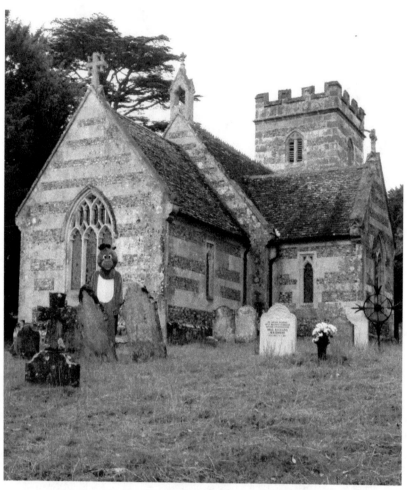

'Where's Will?' This time he's a reindeer outside Chettle church.

114

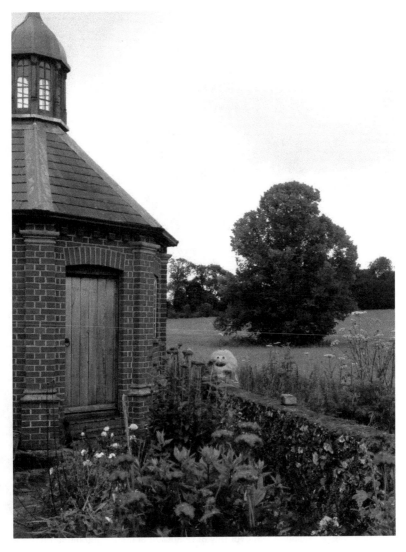

'Where's Will?' Spot the Honey Monster.

no i will

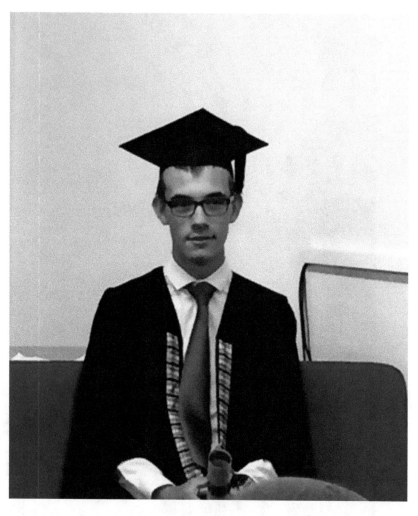

William's last ever day at Beaucroft school, aged nineteen

Chapter Thirteen

I've Been Quiet So The Sun Has Come Out

Towards the end of 2007, Ron was very poorly and in November he was admitted to Bournemouth Hospital suffering with pneumonia. He was eighty-five years old and so understandably everyone was very concerned. The family were all visiting him regularly and we had arranged to go in to see him one Sunday afternoon. Julie had been working at the hotel all morning, and we needed to be ready to leave the moment she returned home from work, but the twins had been really playing up all morning. Despite me laying Will's clothes out on his bed, ten minutes before we were due to leave he walked downstairs dressed as a cow. I have to admit it was a great costume, complete with a full set of udders and a bell, but slightly inappropriate for a hospital visit! Emily seemed to have been blow-drying her hair for an hour, whilst still wrapped in a towel, so I shouted at them and told them if they weren't dressed and ready in five minutes I would make them go in their underwear. It did the trick, and thirty seconds before Julie arrived home we were standing in the kitchen and ready to leave. Julie rushed past us and said she just needed to change quickly as she had got soaked through walking back from the hotel.

Outside it looked like the world was ending; trees were being blown over, the sky was black, and the rain was falling so hard it was bouncing three feet off the ground. I told the children to run as fast as they could to the car and opened the back door and ran out after them. William got to the gate first and, true to form, stood there fumbling with the latch while Emily and I screamed at him to hurry up. I leaned over him, opened the gate, and pushed past and ran to the car whilst unlocking it with the remote key fob. I grabbed the handle and opened the door really fast, whilst ducking down and trying to get in too quickly – and smashed the bridge of my nose on the top corner of the door. I've been punched in the face a thousand times, but this felt like being hit hard with a hammer. I swore loudly and instinctively put my hand to the injury: blood-coloured rain was running through my fingers. I told the children to wait in the car, and ran back to the house to clean my face up – and nearly bumped straight into Julie as she was coming out. She screamed when she saw me, as she said later it looked like I'd been attacked. I grabbed some kitchen roll and told her that she'd better drive, and we headed off to Bournemouth while I sat in the passenger seat with my head bent back and a handful of bloody kitchen roll pressed tightly against my nose.

"That looks bad, does it hurt?" Julie asked.

"No, it's alright," I lied.

"You really are a clumsy twat," whispered Julie and started laughing. The children bravely joined in.

To be fair, she was right, I really am incredibly clumsy, but I have very quick reflexes so I spend my life knocking things over and catching them before they hit the floor!

I checked my face in the vanity mirror and there was a deep one-inch gash across my nose, but I'd managed to stop the bleeding. We got to the hospital, found Ron's ward and pulled up some chairs around his bed. About ten minutes later, I started to get a headache, and my nose was throbbing, so I asked a nurse if I could have a paracetamol. Apparently, they aren't allowed to just administer them without a load of paperwork, so I politely told her not to worry; but two minutes later she returned with a doctor. I told him how I'd done it, which he found very amusing, and after a close look at my nose he confirmed it was broken. I was always proud of the fact that despite years of rugby, martial arts, boxing and sorting the trouble out in pubs no one had ever broken my nose, and then I bloody break it myself getting into my car. Obviously, it was entirely the children's fault!

They say laughter is the best medicine, and it certainly seemed to do the trick for Ron as he made a full recovery!

As Christmas was approaching, Julie offered to organise the children's nativity play in Chettle Church and all of the young children in the village were given a part. They were all handed the script, and the responsibility was on each of them individually to learn their lines as there was only time for one full rehearsal before the play. Emily was the narrator and had lots to read; William was the innkeeper, and the only line he had to remember was, 'There's no room in the inn, but you can have my stable.' For the first few days, the closest he got to getting it right was, 'There's no room, have my stable,' but we persevered for the next two weeks, asking him to repeat the line at every opportunity. We'd ask him to say it first thing in the morning and last thing at night, as he got out of the shower and as he got on his school bus. I used to say it over and over again and get him to repeat it. I even made it tuneful, as he seemed to be able to remember countless song lyrics. I was hearing the bloody line in my head every night I tried to get to sleep: 'There's no room in the inn but you can have my stable' . . . 'there's no room in the inn but you can have my stable'. . . For the last few days before the play he was nailing it, each word spoken clearly and slowly and delivered with great pride, and every time he got it right he would put his hand up for a high-five.

The day of the play arrived and the church was full to brimming with most of the villagers and their families and friends. Some of my family and several friends had come to watch and support the twins and, besides, it was becoming a nice annual tradition getting everyone together and in the Christmas spirit. I had listened to Emily read her lines several times, and apart from encouraging her to slow down she read beautifully. She stood in the vestry and read so eloquently that it was easy to forget you were watching a children's play. Julie was sitting at the front ready to prompt any forgetful children, but they were all remembering and saying their lines perfectly. We waited with baited breath for Will's moment and, when it was time, Julie gave him a big pre-rehearsed nod and he stepped forward with a huge smile on his face, paused for just a second, and then turned back towards his mum and shouted, "What is it again?"

As most of the congregation started giggling, Julie did her best to whisper his words to him and then, with great pride, he said, "There's no inn, have my stable' and took a bow.

When the play was over and everyone was leaving the church all the talk was of William and, despite wonderful performances from all of the children, once again he had stolen the show. Sometimes it really was impossible to know whether William genuinely struggled to get things right, or was doing it purely for comic effect.

After what had felt like the longest countdown in history, finally it was 14th February 2008 and time for us to fly to the Maldives. For Julie and me, this had become so much more than just a holiday, as through all our darkest moments in the five months since that awful incident we had told each other *it's not long now*. All we'd wanted was to escape and be together as a family, where there was nothing to remind us of that time. The twins had never been on such a long flight, but as there were so few children on the plane the crew made a real fuss of them – and Mummy and Daddy were kept in a steady supply of red wine!

The bare-footed pilot of the sea plane let the twins sit up front with him, and for forty minutes we enjoyed the most breath-taking scenery. Below us a myriad of tiny coral islands were sprinkled throughout the sparkling Indian Ocean. The pilot circled the island that would be our home for the next two weeks. He then landed a few hundred yards off the shore and we boarded a small boat that took us to the long wooden jetty. The staff were lined up and singing a traditional welcome song and greeted us with huge smiles, flowers and cocktails. After a quick check in, we were taken to our accommodation, which was a two-bedroomed round wooden thatched villa standing directly on the beach and only fifty yards from the sea. We unpacked as fast as we could and put our swimming costumes on and set off for a walk around the tiny island to explore. After just fifteen minutes we were back where we started, opposite our villa and standing in the crystal blue sea. The brochure hadn't done it justice; it was paradise. We were all holding hands and, as I squeezed Julie's, I said to the children, "What do we say?" and together in unison they threw their arms in the air and shouted, "Aren't we lucky!"

At that very moment, as if on demand, a pod of dolphins surfaced and swam by us along the edge of the reef about fifty yards off shore. Not only was it an amazing sight, but it was strangely emotional, and for Julie and me it felt like a sign that we'd made it, we'd survived, and our family was stronger than ever.

I've always been an early riser and love to walk, so every morning I'd get up before the others and do a couple of laps of the island and watch the sunrise. After a few days, William was just starting to adjust to the time difference, and he woke up when I did and he whispered to me that he wanted to come. I have to be honest, I was reluctant, as he never stopped talking, and I loved the peace and quiet at the start of the day. However, I agreed, and when we were out on the beach and in no danger of waking the girls up I told Will the only way to see the sunrise was to be quiet. I didn't for a minute believe it would work, but we set off on our walk and, to my amazement, he didn't say a single word for half an hour. After two laps we got back to our stretch of beach and sat down with our feet in the water and watched the sun appear from the sea on the horizon. After a while William leaned over and whispered to me, "Look, Daddy, I've been quiet so the sun has come out."

"I know, Will, well done. It's beautiful, isn't it."

"Yes, it is. Daddy, does the sun go away at the end of the day because it's fed up with all the noise?"

I put my arm around him and said, "I think you might be right, Will. Talking of noise, shall we go and wake those bloody women up?"

"Yeah, women, hey," he said, and tutted and rolled his eyes.

Before we'd left England, I'd taken us all to a scuba diving shop near Poole Quay and bought us all snorkels, masks and flippers. My mate Darren had given me some great advice, suggesting I also took with us an inflatable Lilo. Although the children could both swim, to really enjoy the incredible marine life you needed to stay in the water for long periods of time. If I laid the Lilo horizontally in the water, the children could lie vertically across each end, with their masks in the water, and using my flippers I could push from behind and we'd glide around the edge of the reef. It worked perfectly, and with Julie swimming alongside we snorkelled for at least two hours every morning and afternoon. We saw some of the most spectacular coral, thousands of different fish, turtles, manta rays, moray eels, octopus, and even a few sharks. I had an underwater camera strapped to my wrist, and one morning I was snorkelling, pushing the twins along the reef, and I happened to glance up . . . underneath the Lilo the twins were holding hands under the water. I managed to take the shot, and despite countless amazing photos of the incredible marine life that was my favourite photo of all.

After a few days of our holiday we got chatting to a couple who had just arrived, called David and Rachel. They were both headteachers at schools in London and we hit it off straight away. David and I did what Englishmen abroad do and made full use of the all-inclusive facilities. The next day we were nursing our spectacular hangovers around the pool, and David was wearing one of those short white medical ankle socks on one of his feet. William spotted it and swam up to David and, with a look of utter amazement on his face he shouted, "Oh my god, have you fwozen your foot, are you fwosty?"

"Sorry, Will, what do you mean?" said a confused David.

"I said, have you fwozen your foot? You're fwosty, aren't you!" said a now very excited Will.

I explained to David about William's colourful imagination, but nevertheless the name stuck and David was Frosty for the remainder of the holiday. They were only staying for a week, so had to leave before us, so we exchanged contact details and walked with them to the jetty to wave them off. As they were boarding the boat, and we were wishing them a safe trip and promising to keep in touch, William took a step backwards and fell straight off the side of the jetty. It was a ten-foot drop into the sea and the water was very deep there. He immediately disappeared under the water and didn't reappear. I instinctively looked for the bubbles, and jumped further out and managed to come up underneath him and bring him to the surface, the whole thing taking no more than a few seconds. Apart from being a bit tearful, and slightly shaken up, he was completely fine, and Frosty and a couple of the staff bent down and pulled him up onto the jetty. I then raised my arm for a lift up and the staff pulled as hard as they could and got absolutely nowhere. Maldivian men are not the biggest – the guys were probably no more than nine stone each – and I was well over fifteen stone at the time. Frosty tried too, and had little more success.

"We're going to need a crane, yep it's a crane job, anyone got a crane?" Frosty started shouting, much to everyone's amusement.

It also did a great job of diverting Will's attention from what had just happened to him, something I'm sure was no accident on Frosty's part. I managed to climb up myself and, as I stood on the jetty in dripping wet shorts and a T-shirt, laughing at the situation, I then produced from my pocket a soaking wet piece of paper with all their contact details washed away.

"The lengths I'll go to avoid having to keep in touch with you two!" I said sarcastically.

In the absence of a pen and paper, they promised they would contact us when we got home, and true to their word they did and we've remained friends ever since.

The saying in the Maldives is 'No news, no shoes', and I had certainly embraced that philosophy and switched off to the world. When I returned to work it felt like I'd been away forever, and it was one hell of a shock on my first day back to discover the company I worked for was in serious financial difficulties. The country was in a recession, and property is usually the first to take a hit, but I always thought the company would be able to ride the storm. It wasn't the ideal 'welcome home'! In May, just two months later, the company was put into receivership and all of the staff were made redundant.

My boss William had made plans to start another property company, and offered just three of the forty staff the opportunity to go with him – I was one of them. I say 'opportunity'; he was just about broke, so it was a huge risk, but I'd taken them all my life, so nothing new there. For the next few months we achieved so little that the other two staff left and found new jobs. William was finding it very hard to pay my salary, so I agreed to become his business partner and take the risks with him. We explored all sorts of other business opportunities, but kept returning to what we both knew best, eventually conceiving a different way to make money from a desperate property market. There were still many cash-rich people in the area, who were now earning next to no interest on their savings, and there was an abundance of cheap properties to buy that would provide a great rental income. So instead of trying to buy and refurbish or build new houses, we used all our contacts to source cheap properties and supplied them to the investors for a fee. It was slow going in the beginning, but as word spread our success grew and finally I started to earn again.

William and Emma, like us, had their children before they were married, and long before his financial troubles they had arranged to get married in Phuket, Thailand in the October. They had invited us and, at first, I'd declined as we were going to the Maldives. Two extravagant holidays in one year was far too decadent. But then William asked me to be his best man. It was a stretch to afford it, but life's for living so I accepted and booked the four of us to go. Julie and I were really excited about returning to where we'd honeymooned and for the twins to experience Thailand. Although we had an amazing time, it wasn't nearly as easy coping with Will as it had been in the Maldives. He really struggled with the humidity and the food, and I don't think his body clock ever properly adjusted.

Julie and I took it in turns to stay in the room with him in the evenings, until we found out that the hotel offered a child minding service. The first night the child minder turned up we introduced her to William. She was a young Thai girl, and really sweet, and she did her best to explain that she spoke very little English. I told her that she'd get on great with Will as they had something in common, but she didn't get my joke! Halfway through the evening, Julie popped back to the room and Will was fast asleep. The Thai girl was standing directly over his bed, staring at him – it was the hotel's policy in case of any problems with the child in their sleep. Everything was fine, but when we returned to our room a couple of hours later she looked completely traumatised. She was trying to explain what had happened, and was waving her arms around, and after a while we made sense of what she was saying: William had been having his night terrors and she'd learnt some pretty colourful new English words that night.

Although at times it was quite stressful on holiday dealing with a child who didn't really like the heat, late nights or the food, we did have an amazing time. Emily loved every single part of the holiday and Julie and I fell in love with Thailand all over again. The wedding was incredible, but the absolute highlight for us all was swimming with baby elephants. The hotel owned two called Lilly and Lucky, and every afternoon they would be walked down onto the beach and they would run into the sea and take a swim. Although they were babies, they probably still weighed as much as a small car, but were both so gentle and aware of their size. To see William and Emily swimming alongside, laughing and playing with them in the surf, justified the money I'd spent a thousand times over.

Chapter Fourteen

The Bad Conductor Of An Orchestra

In early February 2009, one month before the twins turned twelve, Steve and Emma came to stay for the weekend. They left Derby around lunchtime on the Friday to avoid the worst of the traffic and arrived around four o'clock in the afternoon. We were eating next door in The Castleman that evening, and as no one would have to drive the wine was opened as soon as they walked through the door. We left the twins indoors to watch some television, and the four of us moved up to The Retreat while Steve and I made our standard empty promise to ourselves not to drink like Vikings and ruin our dinner!

After an hour or so Will appeared at the door moaning that Emily wouldn't let him watch what he wanted, but I sent him away and told him that this was adult time. He appeared again, and was sent back to the house. But when he appeared a third time we gave in and let him join us. By now the wine was flowing as well as the conversation and Will wasn't getting the attention he wanted. We hadn't even noticed that he'd turned the music off until out of the blue he started to sing 'Pie Jesu' from Andrew Lloyd Webber's *Requiem*. Our mouths all hit the floor – his voice was absolutely stunning. We listened in stunned silence as he sang the entire song and then proudly took a bow. We gave him a really big round of applause and all asked him to sing it again for us, which he did, very happily. This time I listened really carefully. The lyrics are in Latin, which I was pretty confident William didn't speak, but he'd obviously learned to sing the words as they sounded to him. To be honest, it was difficult to notice the lyrical errors, but he hit every high note with ease. We had absolutely no idea he could sing like that.

When Will had enjoyed enough attention, he walked back to the cottage and Steve looked at us and said, "Well, you two are fucking dark horses, aren't you? You never said he'd been having singing lessons, he's bloody amazing!"

"Yeah, unbelievable. Will's got an incredible voice! How long has he been practising?" said Emma.

"Honestly, we had no clue he could sing like that, we've just heard it for the first time, as you have," I said.

In the spring of the previous year, Britain's Got Talent aired on television for its second series. A young boy called Andrew Johnston walked on stage and very nervously introduced himself and told the judges he got bullied at school because he was in a choir. He sang 'Pie Jesu' so beautifully, and went on to finish third in the final show. We took the twins to watch the live tour when it came to Bournemouth in June, and Andrew was William's favourite performer. Later that year, Andrew Johnston released *One Voice*, his first solo album, and we bought it for William at Christmas. He listened to it in his bedroom all the time, but for those seven weeks before Steve and Emma arrived, we'd not once heard him sing along to it. William was full of surprises but this one knocked us sideways.

We walked back down the garden to the cottage and Julie said to William, "Would you like to sing that in Chettle Church next month in the Mother's Day service? You'll have to practise really hard, would you like that?"

"Yeah, okay. When is next month? Is that the next day?" he said calmly.

For several weeks, he practised all the time and kept getting better. I'm not the kind of father to tell his children they're brilliant when they're not, but his voice was exquisite. On Mother's Day, the church was full, with most of the villagers there, and William was sitting directly in front of me flicking through a Bible. I was actually really nervous for him, but William seemed completely unfazed. As the vicar took his place the congregation fell silent, and at that exact moment Will stood up and turned around towards me, holding the bible, and said really loudly, "Dad, is this that Bible nonsense you were talking about?"

As the usual suspects started giggling, for once in my life I was completely lost for words. I caught the vicar's eye, which only made matters worse, and then glanced towards Roland, who had removed his glasses and was rubbing tears of laughter from his eyes. From behind me I heard someone say, "Out of the mouths of babes," and I quickly motioned for William to sit down whilst I unconsciously slid lower into my pew. For the first time in my life I couldn't wait for a church service to start.

After about fifteen minutes, the vicar introduced William, and I leaned forward and tapped him on the shoulder and told him it was his time to sing. He looked around and very casually said, "Oh, is it? Okay then, Dad," and walked to the front without a care in the world.

As was typical of Chettle Church, the CD hadn't been loaded and there was a couple of minutes of fuss while they worked out how to work a fancy stereo, but it didn't seem to concern Will. Eventually the music for his track started and once again the congregation fell silent. I had heard him sing the song a hundred times by now, but I'd never heard him sing it so beautifully. I allowed myself a glance around the church and not one person noticed me as they were transfixed by William. Everybody knew him and I'm certain they were not expecting what they were hearing. He hit every note effortlessly, and by the time he finished and took his customary bow there wasn't a dry eye in the church. He got a huge round of applause, and as everyone filed out they all congratulated him on his incredible performance. I had never felt so proud in my entire life. It was so good that everyone seemed to have forgotten about his earlier comment. Not one person mentioned it, so I was off the hook too!

It was around this time in his life that I first noticed William had developed a habit of flicking. If he was sitting watching television or listening to music he would always have a pen or a pencil in his hand and would flick it forwards and backwards in the air. He looked a bit like the bad conductor of an orchestra, and at first that's actually what I thought he was trying to mimic. As time went on I realised that it was purely habitual, and although it made him look a little crazy it was better than picking his nose or biting his nails. It did seem to comfort him and so, at first, we didn't interfere. The more worrying habit was when he would become fixated on a tiny scratch or blemish in his skin and he would pick at it until it was red raw or, worse, bleeding. He would moan for days about the tiniest scratch, and worse still a splinter as they would really bother him. Conversely, he seemed to have a very high pain threshold, and we'd seen him have some really bad falls and just get up and brush himself down.

One day we asked Will to go to the village shop and pick up a few things for us. We had an account that we settled once a week so he wouldn't need to deal with money. We'd learned from experience that there was little chance of him remembering more than two items so we would write him a list. He would then just hand it to the shopkeeper, who would get the items for him and put them in a bag. I gave him the small list of about four items and told him he needed to walk down as it was dangerous to go on his scooter and try to carry a bag back. Unfortunately, he ignored me, and on the way back from the shop, with a plastic bag dangling from the handlebars, he lost his balance and fell off. He left his scooter on the side of the road and walked back to our cottage, and seemed more worried about being told off for taking his scooter than the fact that he was cut, bruised and bleeding.

For the next few days he drove us mad complaining about a scratch on his finger. It was so small but so typical of William to be bothered about it. He kept saying it hurt and we kept telling him to stop fussing about it. He would sit in his armchair just staring at it, and then look at us as if we were the most horrible parents in the world not to take this tiny scratch seriously. After a few days, I happened to notice his fingers were swollen and so I took a closer look – and he'd clearly broken two of his fingers, which the doctor later confirmed. You can imagine how shit we felt. For days he'd been fixating on a scratch as if that was the cause of the pain, and in the absence of any initial swelling we had no idea it was anything more serious. I took some comfort from the fact that my mum and dad had failed to notice my brother Pete's broken fingers when he was a young boy! But Julie and I were certainly not going to win any parenting prizes that year!

Since the beginning of the year Henry's health had been deteriorating rapidly. He was nearly fifteen years old, which is a very good age for a Labrador, and the visits to the vets were becoming ever more frequent. Our walks were now limited to a slow walk around one field, and I came back one day and told Julie I didn't think he had much longer. We were broken-hearted. Like most elderly Labs, he was suffering from arthritis, and his hearing and eyesight were now very poor. He was nearly two years old when the twins were born, and had been part of our family for all of their lives. I asked the children to come into the dining room, and I explained how poorly Henry was and that he may not have much longer to live. Emily just stood up and wrapped her arms around me and told me how sorry she was, and then laid down and cuddled Henry in his bed. William didn't really understand the reality of the situation and thought I was teasing him.

"He's not going to die, Daddy, you're joking, aren't you? I'm not going to die, am I?"

"Everybody dies eventually, Will, but you don't have to worry about that, you'll live for a very long time. Now you just have to be very gentle around Henry. He's a very old man and he needs lots of rest. Just give him lots of love."

"No I will," said William.

The next day Julie took William with her to go shopping in Blandford – she always bought our meat from the local butchers in the town, and all the guys who work there really looked forward to seeing William every week as he always made them laugh.

He walked in ahead of Julie, and all of the butchers smiled and greeted him warmly and the manager said, "Hey, Will mate, how you doing? Good to see you."

"Do you know what? My dog Enwy is dying, he's really big, and if you want you can have all his meat to sell. You can have his legs and his body and put them here in your counter."

Julie grabbed Will's hand, spun him around and said, "William, don't be so horrible, we don't eat dogs and you love Henry, don't you!"

"Yeah, but it is meat, isn't it? I wouldn't mind. My mates can have him."

There was an element of him showing off and deliberately trying to be funny, but it also proved he wasn't able to comprehend how he would feel when the inevitable happened. When I was the same age as the twins our family dog Chico, who was also a black Labrador, had to be put down, and I can still remember that day clearly and how upset I was.

Henry and I had been inseparable for nearly fifteen years; we'd walked thousands and thousands of miles together in every kind of weather. When I had the car showroom he came to work with me every day; before I could afford staff, he was often the only company I had for days on end. My children had learned to walk by holding onto him. He'd moved with us from house to house, and wherever I was sitting he would be next to me. Although he loved Julie and the twins, the bond between us was so strong. He was so loyal and I knew he would've given his life to protect me.

I laid on the floor next to his bed for hours one night, and his breathing was so poor I knew I'd have to make that call to the vets the following morning. (Fortunately, with our pets we can decide when they've suffered enough.) It was the end of May, and the children were on half-term, so before the vet arrived our niece Megan came and got the children and took them down the road. After a quick examination, he said the kindest thing to do was to put him to sleep. Julie and I cuddled Henry as the injection was administered and the vet respectfully left the moment he took his last breath. We completely broke down.

When we'd finally stopped crying I wrapped him in a sheet and his favourite blanket and picked him up to carry him to the end of our garden. I was adamant that I would hold it together in front of the children, but as I was carrying him I started crying again, just as they walked through the gate. It hadn't occurred to me that they had never once in their lives seen me cry. William looked really confused and kept repeating, "Daddy, why you cryning? Please stop cryning, please stop cryning," as he sobbed and rubbed at my arm.

Henry's favourite place to lie was under an apple tree next to The Retreat at the end of the garden. My best mate Darren and his three children, Sophie, Isabelle and Louis, had given us the tree a year before as a thank you for having them all to stay, and we'd planted it together. I dug his grave next to the tree, and when I'd buried him Julie and the twins came up to say their goodbyes. Emily was upset because she knew she'd never see Henry again, but it was the sight of me crying that was haunting William. Later that evening I was sitting on Will's bed with him and I told him that it's okay for men to cry; we don't cry if we hurt ourselves, but if we are upset then it's okay to cry.

"You're not upset now though, Daddy, are you? You won't cry anymore, will you?" Will said, and put his arms around me and squeezed me tight.

I said, "No, Will, not anymore, you've made me better."

We always knew we would get another dog; it was only a question of when. I'm not sure what the correct amount of grieving time is, but our house felt empty without one. For the next few weeks we deliberated about it until we felt we couldn't be without a dog for any longer. We knew we wouldn't get another Labrador, as there would never be another Henry and, after much researching, we decided a Boxer would be perfect for our family. They are wonderful with children, love exercise, are very affectionate and, despite some negative press, are very intelligent dogs.

I spent ages looking on the internet for the country's top breeders and found a lady who not only bred championship Boxers but was also a judge at Crufts. Her dogs were beautiful, and I wrote to her expressing our desire to meet her and potentially buy one of her puppies. I was incredibly disappointed when she replied telling me she wouldn't sell to anyone who'd never had a Boxer before. I was so frustrated, but decided to persevere and wrote to her again saying that I completely understood and respected her stance but I knew we'd be able to give a wonderful home to any dog. Thankfully she replied and put me in touch with another breeder, who was a friend of hers, and had used one of her championship dogs as a stud and just had a litter of eight. Due to a change in circumstances there were three puppies still looking for a home. The only problem was she lived in Inverness! I had long chats with her on the telephone, and she sent me countless photographs of her dogs and many testimonials from other previous buyers – the pedigree of the puppies was exceptional. Reassuringly, she asked me loads of questions about our home and our experience with dogs. I sent her loads of photos of Chettle and our cottage and she was delighted that one of her puppies would have such a nice life. We are always told not to buy a dog on the internet, but I knew I'd been as thorough as one could be and couldn't have done any more research.

After studying the fifty photos she sent me of the puppies we chose our dog. He was red with a big splash of white on his chest, a jet-black face, four white paws and big thoughtful eyes. She asked me what name she should put on his collar and I told her George. Every couple of days she would send us more photos of him and we were already very much in love. When he was finally ready to leave his mum, we arranged to meet her at her son's house in Coventry and tied it in with an overnight stay in Derby with Steve and Emma. We were so excited, but there was that tiny niggling worry that we were taking a risk buying a puppy we hadn't met from people we didn't know. We needn't have worried, from the first moment we set eyes on George we knew we'd hit the jackpot. He was the most beautiful puppy I'd ever seen and he immediately ran to Julie and me and started rolling around at our feet. It was love at first sight for the three of us.

We went back to our car and got his travel cage – we'd put soft blankets and some toys in it. The lady put in a small towel that smelt of George's mum and we set off for home. We stopped several times on the journey back, and George walked happily next to us on his lead and did a wee when asked. If anyone else told me this I would find it hard to believe, but I swear George came to us already trained.

He seemed to be able to read my mind and instinctively did whatever I was thinking. We phoned ahead and asked June to make sure the twins were waiting in the garden. When we got home I carried him through the gate and said to the twins, "Will, Emily, I'd like you to meet George."

I put him down and he ran to the twins and rolled around on the grass with them, licking their faces. It was the middle of summer and I'd taken a week off work to spend every moment with him.

Later that day I was sitting on The Retreat steps with a glass of wine in my hand, and William was lying on the grass under the apple tree cuddling George and I heard him whisper, "George, this is where Enwy is buwied. My Daddy loved him but he loves you now and he won't be upset anymore. Enwy was my bruvver, but now you are my bruvver."

Chapter Fifteen

What Do I Wear?

M y best mate Darren had served with the Royal Marines for seventeen years, having joined shortly after leaving school. In 2004, he left and took a post as a contract officer for the United Arab Emirates Marines and emigrated to Dubai with his wife and three very young children, Sophie, Isabelle and Louis. It was Darren's second marriage, and he had two children from his first, Jack and Hannah. Sadly, after three years in Dubai, his wife told him the marriage was over and she moved back to Wimborne with the children, leaving Darren to complete his posting in Dubai. Naturally, he was broken-hearted. Over the next few months I was on the phone to him constantly, and just when he'd promised me that he was okay and I could stop worrying about him, I had to make the hardest phone call I've ever made in my life. Darren's first-born son Jack had been killed in a car crash; he was only eighteen-years-old and I had to break the news to him.

Our friendship was extremely strong. Since we were five years old we had always had each other's backs and there was nothing we wouldn't do for each other. Darren had a really tough childhood. His mum treated him like a lodger in her house, even as a young boy, and his stepfather was a bully. He would avoid being at home as much as possible, so if we weren't at mine, we would spend hours just walking our dogs around Wimborne. As a teenager, he started to train really hard so he could join the Royal Marines and was the fittest boy in school. After he had completed his first three months in the Marines, he had some leave and called his house when he got off the train at Poole to get a lift home. When he couldn't get through he phoned someone else, who then informed him his mum and stepfather had moved to Wales – they hadn't even told him. He was only seventeen. Darren is now a big guy, and as strong as an ox; he has a wicked sense of humour and his round, kind face belies the hard-as-nails character that he is.

Whenever Darren was able to fly home I let him stay in The Retreat so that he would have somewhere he could be with his children – fortunately, Julie, Will and Emily loved him to bits too. His children were amazing, and got on really well with ours, even though there was quite an age gap. The twins were twelve, and Sophie, Isabelle and Louis were seven, six and five respectively in the summer of 2009, when they were coming to stay. Apart from our big garden with the swimming pool and trampoline, Chettle was one giant playground for the children and they could play around the village all day. Of course, we also had an adorable puppy that would keep them entertained for hours. I couldn't wait to see them all and we were getting everything ready for their arrival.

I own a sit-on tractor mower and was about to cut the grass when William started pleading with me to let him do it. Over the previous few years he had progressed from sitting on my lap while I drove it, to having the odd go on his own while I supervised very carefully! He was desperate to do it, and since I had lots more to be getting on with I gave in and said yes. We could put up with strange patterns in the grass for a week! His face lit up and he jumped up and down with excitement.

"Fanks, Dad, fank you so much, oh my god, I am so happy, I'll twy and do stwaight lines like you do. Fank you, fank you so much, Daddy."

"Okay, Will, just be very careful, and always look where you're going," I said.

"No I will. Daddy, what do I wear?" he asked, as if there was some correct grass-cutting attire.

"Anything you want," I said, without giving it any thought.

It was a particularly hot day in August, so I went up to The Retreat to open all the windows and finish getting it ready for Darren and his children. Ten minutes later I heard the mower start. I looked down the garden and driving towards me was Will, concentrating really hard and dressed as Father Christmas. He even had the big white beard on!

"Is dis okay, Daddy? Am I doing a good job? Are you improud of me?" he shouted over the noise of the mower.

I was laughing so much I hadn't heard Darren's car pull up, and suddenly the gate flew open and the three children came charging into the garden shouting "WILLIAM!" followed by Darren carrying several bags. I ran down to greet them and help with the bags and George ran to the children and rolled around at their feet.

"Hey, Mr M, any reason why Will's dressed as Father Christmas?" asked Darren.

"Well, he asked me what he should wear and I said, 'anything you want'."

"Fair one," said Darren. "Nice pretty patterns too. Is he on LSD?" He laughed and gave me one of his huge man-hugs.

Later that evening we were sitting around the fire-pit, enjoying yet another bottle of wine, when Darren told me he had some news: he'd got himself a new job. He was leaving Dubai and going to work in another country. It was on a rotation basis so he'd be able to come back every couple of months and asked if he could use The Retreat when he did.

I said, "Of course, that's fantastic news, you'll get to see your children more regularly now."

"Yeah, I know. I'm really chuffed, and you can always come and stay with me if you fancy a break from Chettle. It's in Kabul, Afghanistan," he smiled.

"How lovely for you, I'll think about it. Yep, I've thought about it . . . get fucked!" I said.

A couple of days later I suggested that Darren and I took all five children up to the woods to collect some kindling. It was good to fill the wood shed with dry kindling in the summer ready for all those winter fires. We grabbed some sacks and borrowed the Estate's pick-up truck. I drove, and Darren and all the children sat in the open cargo bed at the back holding on to the sides. I drove up to the woods, and after an hour or so we had several large sacks of kindling. They all climbed back into the truck and I shouted out of the window, "Is everybody ready? Hold on tight."

"Yes, we're weady, go weally fast," shouted a very excited William.

The pick-up truck isn't capable of going fast, but to give them some fun I accelerated quickly. Immediately all the children started shouting "Stop!" I pulled over, confused as to what the problem was, and looked in the wing mirror. There was a huge cloud of dust, and as it settled Darren appeared through the cloud, a big bear of a man hobbling up the track.

"You alright, mate, what happened to you?" I asked.

"I was about to take a photo of all the kids, next minute Will's shouted go and I'm somersaulting out the back of the bloody pick-up. Nice one, Mr M, I've worked all over the world in some of the biggest hell-holes on earth and you nearly kill me in Chettle!"

He'd had his finger on the camera button and had taken several photos of the sky as he'd somersaulted backwards out of the van. The children thought it was hysterical.

We loved having children to stay, but the only problem was William would always become the age of the youngest child present. Whatever allowances were made, for example, for a five-year-old Louis, William would expect the same, and get very frustrated if we expected any more from him. Although I was very happy for William to be so free-spirited, and dress up in all his costumes, I still desperately wanted him to grow up. It was a constant battle between letting him be himself and wanting my boy to become a young man. Although they were very rare, any rows between Julie and me would invariably be about her treating him like a little boy. It was certainly not only Julie though. It felt to me that as hard as I was trying to help Will to grow up, there were too many people who seemed to forget Will was nearly a teenager and treated him like a toddler. Like anyone, the more you do for them the less they will do for themselves. It was my biggest frustration, and it always felt that as I tried to take William a few steps forward, he would be dragged back by well-meaning people. I'm the first to admit, however, that Julie is the real hero in our family and if I spent as much time with William as she did, I'm sure I too would do anything to make a day go smoother.

I had a brilliant relationship with Emily. It's fair to say she was a real daddy's girl, and she always affectionately referred to us as 'the A-Team'. We were very similar and, like me at school, was no academic, but she was very smart. She understood people and from a young age she had a very intuitive mind. She loved spending time with me, and I tried to teach her the stuff that isn't taught at school; life lessons like having integrity, not procrastinating, trusting your instincts, setting goals, learning to enjoy mistakes, challenging yourself and, above all, laughing at yourself. I really enjoyed our conversations, and I hoped that we would still have a great relationship when she turned thirteen, as all too often children become teenagers and inexplicably decide their parents are complete twats.

Emily was having horse-riding lessons from a friend in the village and desperately wanted her own horse. In principal, I liked the idea of it; better she was in Chettle taking care of her horse rather than wanting constant lifts to town to just hang around with her friends. However, I needed an awful lot of convincing that it wasn't just a fad and she fully understood the size of the commitment. For several months she pleaded with me, but I refused every time. Secretly, though, I'd had discussions with June and she was prepared to give up a barn and one of her paddocks for a horse if needed.

In September 2009, after twenty years of membership at Broadstone Golf Club, I left and joined a relatively new golf course called Remedy Oak. It was only ten minutes from Chettle and one of the best courses I had ever played. As the children were growing up, I was lucky if I got to play once a week, but my handicap at the time was six and I loved the sport. I'd always hoped to be able to play more golf as the children got older, and I could now see an opportunity to do that. Julie was interested in getting back into riding, so if I bought a horse suitable for all the family they would be more than happy if Daddy disappeared to the golf course more often!

One evening, when Julie was at work and William had gone to bed, Emily and I were having a chat in the dining room. She brought up the subject of getting a horse again and I told her she had no idea how much work would be involved. As far as she was concerned I was completely against the idea. But she fought her corner like a seasoned barrister in a courtroom. Every barrier I put up she knocked down, and she was passionate and very convincing. I made her fight for what she wanted for over an hour, just to make absolutely sure I wouldn't be making a mistake. Eventually, I was all out of questions, and she looked exhausted, so I took a deep breath, stood up and said, "Okay, Emily, I believe you, we'll get a horse."

"Dad, please don't joke about this, are you serious, do you mean it?" she said, and her eyes immediately filled with tears.

"Yes, Emily, I am. I just needed to make sure you were serious. Promise me you'll include William and won't have too many arguments with your mum – she knows more about horses than you do."

She ran around the table and threw her arms around me and said, "I promise, I promise."

A few days later I was chatting to an old friend of mine I knew from my days in the motor trade. Alan is what you would describe as a 'loveable rogue' and had several business interests, one of which was race horses. I told him I was looking for a horse for Emily and he told me I could have one of his.

Alan leaned back in his chair and said, "It's never done any bloody good, mate, useless thing has never won a race, you can have it."

I was really happy and phoned Julie and told her I'd found Emily a horse, it was called Lauren's Treasure, and Alan was going to give it to me for nothing.

Julie said, "Richard, you bloody idiot, that's a race horse, Emily would be thrown off and killed in seconds. We need an old bombproof pony. You really know nothing about horses, do you. I think we'll leave the searching to me."

For the next few months and into 2010 she searched, without success. All the good ones were either sold really quickly or far more money than we were prepared to pay. We were going to Thailand again in February, with the children and Steve and Emma, so Julie decided they would continue the search when we got back. As is often the case, the moment they decided to wait an advert appeared for the perfect pony. It was an hour's drive away, and Julie asked me to go along with them in case there was any negotiating to do. The young couple who were selling the pony were really lovely and Julie, Will and Emily fell in love with Prince. Emily rode him around their yard, and even though I knew nothing about horses it was clear that they were a perfect match. The couple were desperately sad to be selling him, but needed the money towards a deposit for their first house so I decided not to quibble on the price. We agreed to pick him up upon our return from Thailand.

We had long discussions with William before we booked to go to Phuket again, as he wasn't keen on the food or the heat, but he assured us he wanted to go. Steve and Emma understood him very well, and with them there to support us we had one of our best ever holidays. William was so much happier this time, and by making sure he took a nap each day he was able to stay up with us every evening. We went out on a speed boat and ate at a floating restaurant. We kayaked through sea caves, went on tuk-tuk rides into Patong, and Will and Emily had their first Thai massages on the beach. Once again, the highlight was when we took a taxi back to the hotel we'd stayed at previously and we all got to swim in the sea with the elephants, Lilly and Lucky.

We arrived home, and just two days later Julie went with a friend who owned a horse box and collected Prince and brought him back to Chettle. Although I'd given Emily a tough time over getting a horse, she really deserved this. Having a twin brother like William can't have been easy for her. We expected a lot from her, and I was painfully aware that William took up a far bigger share of our time, yet she

no I will

never complained. I was extremely proud of her, and what daddy, if he could, wouldn't want to make his daughter's dreams come true.

Chapter Sixteen

Rest In Pieces

O n 12th March 2010 the twins turned thirteen and the dreaded teenage years began. I was quietly confident that William would not turn into a stroppy teenager any time soon, and hoped that with Emily's focus being on Prince we may've delayed the inevitable with her for at least some time. Although emotionally and intellectually William was years behind, physically he was like most other thirteen-year-old boys and he hit puberty around this time. For most teenagers, the changes their bodies go through can be the cause of great embarrassment and worry, but not for Will, as he had no insecurities and certainly wasn't body-conscious.

One Sunday morning, William and Emily and her friend Maddie were sitting around the dining room table eating breakfast. Maddie was Emily's best friend, she'd stayed over, and the three of them were all going to go out for the morning with Prince and George. I was ironing a golf shirt in readiness for a game at Remedy Oak, when out of the blue William put his knife and fork down and said, "Daddy, do you know what? I'm getting hairs on my funny things, you know, my balls," and pulled his pyjama bottoms out and pointed to them as if we needed some indication as to where his testicles were.

Maddie cracked up and Emily immediately turned bright red and shouted, "Oh my god, William, you are so embarrassing!"

"William, that's not appropriate to talk about at breakfast, and certainly not in front of the girls," I said, as sternly as I could while doing my best to suppress a laugh.

"Is it not? Well, it's twue though, I'm getting hairy balls like a man, like you!" he said proudly.

"Okay, we get it, Will. Enough now. I'll talk to you about it later, you're embarrassing your sister."

"I will not take you with us today if you say things like that, William. Oh my god, Daddy, why has he got to be such an idiot?" shouted Emily.

"Don't call him an idiot, Emily, be nice to each other. And William, I don't want to hear later that you've said anything else inappropriate. You need to be a gentleman, okay?"

"Okay, but can I show you them later?" he asked, and nodded in their direction.

"Oh, for god's sake, this family is like so embarrassing!" Emily screamed, and stormed out of the room.

"I'm sorry about that, Maddie, did you enjoy your breakfast?" I asked.

"I did thank you, and don't worry, that's the most fun I've had at breakfast for a long time," she said, with a big smile.

The girls got dressed much quicker than William, who was taking an eternity, and soon enough Emily was shouting at him again about how slow he was and how he was ruining their day. Normally I would've insisted they got on, but I did feel for Emily, so I asked Will if he wanted to come to golf with me instead. Will's absolute favourite thing to do was to drive a golf buggy. I'd always walked when I played golf, but since I'd joined Remedy Oak now and again I would play on my own and let Will drive me around the course. He found it almost impossible to stay quiet, and many a time he would start talking in the middle of my swing only for me to slice my ball into a lake – much to his amusement. This day I had arranged a game with three of my friends, so on the way to the club I drummed it into him about how important it was to stay still and be quiet whenever somebody was playing a shot. I emphasised the importance of good behaviour and respecting the other players so much that I felt sure he'd understood.

We got to the clubhouse and I explained to Lee, Scott and Rich why I had Will with me and, as expected, they were all more than happy for him to come around with us. I promised them he knew how to behave and wouldn't put them off.

We partnered up and while Will sat very still and quietly in the buggy we all hit our first tee shots. Lee's went left, Scott's went high and right, and Rich topped his. I was the last to play and happened to hit it really well down the middle of the fairway. As soon as I'd hit my ball William got out of the buggy and approached us all on the tee and said very loudly, "Excuse me, guys, but my daddy is much better than you."

"William, what did I say? Be polite and show respect. Sorry lads," I said, smiling.

"Don't tell him that, Will, his head won't fit back in the buggy," said Scott, and Will started laughing.

Although William was pretty good and managed to stay quiet for most of the time, we soon realised any chance of a serious game had gone out of the window. The lads all have a great sense of humour, and Will was making them laugh telling them all about his hairy balls. Several holes later we were driving down a path, and ahead of us Lee was walking and carrying his golf bag across his back. I told Will to steer around him and turned around in my seat to get a jumper. The next thing I know I felt the impact as the front right side of our buggy collided with the left side of Lee's golf bag. Will slammed the brakes on, and I was thrown forwards into the windscreen and instinctively shouted, "Fuck me!" I glanced right and Lee was spinning in a complete circle, just about managing to stay on his feet.

"Oh my god, Daddy I did dat! Sowry mate, sowry Lee, are you alwight?" said a panicked Will.

"Yeah, I'm okay, Will, don't worry. Bloody hell, Matthews, is there anything you won't do to win a match?" said Lee.

William was genuinely worried and wouldn't stop going on about it. He thought he would be in big trouble with the golf club. I told him to forget about it, there was no damage whatsoever to the buggy so there was no need to mention it. As soon as we finished though he jumped out of the buggy, ran straight up to the head professional Nigel and shouted, "Excuse me, oh my god, do you know what? I crashed the buggy into Lee, I'm bery, bery sowry. My Dad said I shouldn't tell you though. Am I in big twouble?"

Luckily, I'd known Nigel for about twenty-five years, and he was very familiar with stories of William's antics. He told him there was nothing to worry about, and while Will used the toilet I told Nigel what had happened and what Will had said at the breakfast table.

"You're having a great day then aren't you, Rich, did you manage to play well?" said Nigel.

I smiled and said, "No, I played like a wanker. Kind of tough to concentrate with Will around."

I tried on many occasions to teach William how to play golf, and nothing would've given me greater pleasure than playing my favourite sport with my son. If you've never played golf, trust me, it's extremely difficult to do, let alone well, and William found it nearly impossible. It takes incredible coordination, and if I took Will to the driving range where he could just swing away at a ball, he'd miss it nine times out of ten. He'd get frustrated quickly and, just like when I'd tried to teach him to box, he would forget what I taught him and lose interest fast. On the very odd occasion, where he managed to make contact with the golf ball, he was really happy, but then his frustrations would escalate when he couldn't do it again. Whenever we went Julie would wish me luck, and as soon as we walked back through the door she'd ask if it was any better this time. She knew how much it meant to me, and although I always put a brave face on it she could tell how much it upset me.

Although there was no overnight change in William, as time went on he became far more challenging to deal with. Although his extra chromosome made a huge difference to him, it wasn't that alone that made him who he was; he was his father's son, and many of his character flaws were just the worst bits of me. He was starting to show signs of aggression. Whereas in the past if something was too challenging for him he'd just cry or give up, now he was swearing and shouting. It could be the simplest thing, like trying to put his shoes on, and you'd hear him shout 'For fuck's sake!' followed by the sound of shoes hitting the wall, immediately followed by a 'Sowry, Dad'.

Arguments between him and Emily became more frequent, as he was no longer prepared for her to be his boss and he started answering back to his mum or disobeying her completely. Consequently, my role evolved into the scary dad. 'Just wait until your dad gets home,' Julie would say on an almost daily basis. Luckily it worked for her every time, and immediately he'd apologise and plead with her not to tell me. She would assure him that she wouldn't, his behaviour would improve, and then the second I walked through the door he'd tell me anyway. He could never keep anything to himself, even if it got him into trouble.

Although none of it was too bad, the aggression was my biggest concern. I got into loads of fights at school, usually because I was protecting the weak and sometimes, to my detriment, because I was never able to walk away from a challenge. I would never start it, though, so at least I could always justify my actions. My biggest fear was William not being able to control himself, hurting someone, and having no comprehension of the consequences of his actions.

One day, in the summer holidays, Darren had some leave and was staying in The Retreat with his three children. I was at work and William's behaviour had been pushing everyone's patience to the limits. Julie was ironing some clothes in the dining room ready for them to go out together and she heard the twins arguing upstairs. The argument was escalating quickly and they were shouting at each other as they came downstairs. They were obviously not aware their mum was in the house due to the language they were both using, and then she heard Emily shout, "William, don't hurt me, how dare you!"

She then shoved him so hard that he went the length of our dining room and crashed into my trophy cabinet breaking one of the glass doors – she was still much stronger than he was. Julie went ballistic, and any plans of a nice day out together got cancelled and the twins were sent to their rooms for the remainder of the day. She phoned me and gave me the heads-up so I wouldn't arrive home to a nasty surprise. When I got home, instead of doing what they would've expected and going straight upstairs and shouting at them both, I left it for another hour or so. The apprehension would be far worse for them. I sat on The Retreat steps with Darren, watching his children play in the garden with George.

"So, how are you going to play this one, Mr M? I bet they're shitting a brick upstairs. I'm fucking scared for them! Of all things, it had to be your bloody trophy cabinet, didn't it! We'd have got a proper hiding off our dads, wouldn't we?"

"That's for sure. I'm going to make them stew for a while longer and then I think I'll play the disappointed card. I reckon there's been enough shouting in this house for one day. You know, act all sad and stuff, I can't believe you guys are fighting, I've brought you up to love each other, and so on. The problem is, William won't always be the weaker one, and he has to know he can't hurt girls. I think for now the shock of what happened has probably done the job, but if it happens again I'll have to come down on him like a ton of bricks."

It did work, and our nice family life was restored for a while. However, just a few weeks later I was sitting on the sofa in the lounge, and Julie and Will were in the dining room at the opposite end of the cottage. From where I was sitting I could see Julie. William had his back to me and she was attempting to squeeze one of his spots – one of the delights of having a teenage boy! William was very nearly as tall as his mum now, and his voice was starting to break. She obviously hurt him a bit and he shouted really aggressively, and lunged forward and grabbed her around the neck. I saw the shock on her face, and was out of my chair and across the hallway in the blink of an eye. Before he even knew what was happening I'd grabbed him by his jumper with both hands and picked him up off the floor so his eyes were level with mine. With his feet off the ground I shouted at him at the top of my voice, like a drill instructor reprimanding a new recruit. He would never have seen me look so angry, but it was completely orchestrated: although I was cross I deliberately went over the top to put the fear of God into him.

I am very aware that there are many other ways to have dealt with it, and I'm sure some people will think I should've sat him down and gently explained the error of his ways, but I know my son, and I knew what had to be done. I didn't enjoy scaring him one bit, but right then he needed a short, sharp shock. Later that day, when everything had calmed down, we talked for ages about the qualities that real tough men have. I told him it has nothing to do with size or muscles, it's the willingness to do what no one else will. To carry on regardless of the size of the challenge, to withstand hardship and to never give up. I told him no real man ever hurts a girl; real men stand up to bullies and protect those weaker than them.

Several weeks later Julie got a call from Will's teacher, and after the initial pleasantries, she said, "Mrs Matthews, the reason I'm calling you is to let you know what happened today at school. There was a group of about five boys from St Michael's Middle School hanging around outside our school gate and they were picking on one of our younger students. He was clearly very intimidated and was getting quite upset. The teacher on duty in the playground had just noticed what was going on, and was going over to move the boys on. He then saw William marching towards them and, apparently, he gave them all a piece of his mind. Now please don't worry, he is not in any trouble at all. In fact, according to my colleague, he was very impressive and he sent all five boys off with their tails between their legs."

That evening I told him how proud I was of him and asked him if he was scared at the time. He said he wasn't, because bullies were just cowards. Maybe the apple hadn't fallen so far from the tree after all.

Although I had many reservations about getting Emily a horse it was working out really well. All her time was taken up looking after Prince and it was having a really positive effect on her. For the first time in her life she had full responsibility of caring for an animal, and with that and her school homework she was a busy girl. William was fundamentally a lazy boy and liked nothing more than coming home from school and plonking himself down on the sofa in front of the television. He would never volunteer to do anything; but, to his credit, he would never moan or complain if we asked him to do something. It could be walking George or emptying the dishwasher, or just tidying his room, but as soon as we asked he'd just say okay and do it. However, having seen the difference in Emily, we knew we needed to find something to occupy Will's time and give him some responsibility.

I came home from work one day and Julie said she'd been talking with her mum, and she had suggested getting some chickens for Will. At first, I said it was a terrible idea, he wouldn't look after them and it would end up as just another responsibility for us. Julie said I may well be right, but thought we should at least give him the chance – at the very least we'd have our own eggs. Behind The Retreat at the end of our garden, Ron and June had some land where he could keep them, and he would have to feed them, top up their water bowls, clean them out and collect the eggs. June was prepared to help with stuff like de-fleaing and John, the farmer in the village, had an old chicken coop that we could have that just needed a fresh coat of paint. They'd obviously put a lot of thought into this, so I agreed, and we asked William if he'd like his own chickens. Naturally, he was very excited. Kevin and Rose lived at the other end of the village and had a lot of chickens – they were all ex-battery hens – and once we got the coop ready and all the fencing done they kindly gave William six for himself.

He was like a kid at Christmas for the first couple of weeks. He gave them all names, ranging from the normal to the obscure. We had a Wendy, a Wilma, a SpongeBob and even a Parachute. The names seemed to change daily, but his favourite was Parachute. He topped up their water regularly, fed them, cleaned them out and, when they laid an egg, you'd think he'd won the lottery. He'd come running down the garden holding an egg in the air like it was the Olympic torch! I told Will that when we had enough for our family he could sell the rest around the village and the money would be his. We had several egg boxes ready for him, and I explained that when one box was full – that was six eggs – he could sell them to the villagers for one pound. Later that day I saw him run out of our gate with just one egg in his hand. I shouted after him and he said he was selling it to Jonathan, a neighbour who lived just the other side of the hotel. Shortly after he returned with a huge smile on his face, his first business deal done. He had six pounds in his hand.

I smiled and said, "Will, mate, have you just sold Jonathan one egg for six pounds? It's supposed to be six eggs for one pound! Was he happy?"

"Yes, Daddy, he was very happy. He said he wants more when I get them."

"I bet he does," I said.

I phoned Jonathan and apologised that my son had ripped him off. He laughed and told me he didn't want to upset Will, so just drop some down whenever we had more than we needed.

Emily soon realised that her entrepreneurial brother was making some money and felt left out, so I told her she needed to think of a way she could make money from Prince. I already had an idea but wanted her to come up with it on her own. A couple of days later she walked into our bedroom in the morning and said, "Dad, do you think people would buy Prince's shit for their gardens?"

I laughed at her choice of words, but was pleased she'd worked it out for herself. "I reckon they would, you could put a poster on the Chettle noticeboard," I said. "If I were you, though, I'd probably put 'Well-Rotted Horse Manure for Sale'. I think that sounds better than horse shit!"

So, for a while, Emily was delivering wheelbarrows full of horse manure around the village at one pound a barrow. And Will was robbing our neighbours of their hard-earned cash for eggs at whatever price he dreamed up on the day.

It wasn't long before one of Will's chickens got poorly and died – they were probably quite old before we got them, and this one's health had been slowly deteriorating. William was really upset and wanted me to dig a hole and bury it next to Henry. I did it for him, and as we covered it over I asked him if he wanted to say a few words.

No I will

With tears in his eyes he bowed his head and said, "I love you, Parachute, rest in pieces."

I said, "Will, that's really sweet, but it's rest in peace, not pieces."

"No, Daddy, you're wrong. Rest in pieces, like chicken pieces," he said, with absolute conviction.

I smiled and said, "Sorry, mate, my mistake, I think your version is much better."

A few days later I heard him calling one of his chickens Parachute so I said, "Will, we buried Parachute last week, have you forgotten that he died?"

In a completely monotone voice he said, "No, Dad, but I like the name so now this one's Parachute."

Chapter Seventeen

George Wants To Talk To You

I remember my first day at Queen Elizabeth Comprehensive School as if it was yesterday. It's a huge school in Wimborne that takes in students from the age of thirteen from four different middle schools, and each year may have as many as four to five hundred students. Emily had completed four years at Cranborne Middle School, and in September 2010 she started at Q.E, twenty-six years after my first day there. It can be quite daunting for any child but Emily took it all in her stride and enjoyed her first day.

William had completed three years with the same class at Beaucroft and was moving up into the seniors. For the first time, he was going to have a male teacher and Julie and I were delighted. I couldn't fault any of his previous teachers at Beaucroft, but away from school there was no doubt that William responded and behaved better for men, so I was confident it would be the same in class. Will's new teacher was Duncan Russell and the first time I met him I knew that he'd do wonders with William. He had a fantastic sense of humour and clicked with Will straight away. The classroom assistant teacher was Sally Blythe (she was lovely), and together her and Duncan were a great team. He would be in their class for three years and I genuinely felt for the first time that William had every chance of doing the very best that he could do.

Analysing William's progress at school was always difficult. There was some progress year on year, but not in the core subjects upon which a student would normally be judged. As far as I could tell, there had been absolutely no improvement in his reading or writing, and he had little or no comprehension of mathematics. This is no slur on the school, it's just that William wasn't improving despite several different approaches to the teaching methods. At Beaucroft they recognise every child is unique, and the syllabus reflects each child's abilities and needs, and the plan for William going forward was to include as much real-life experience as possible into his education. For example, he would have to create a shopping list from a recipe, they would go to the shops where he would have to find those ingredients, use money to pay, then bring the ingredients back to school and cook the meal.

Once every term there was a parents' evening, where we would meet with his teachers to discuss his progress. Because William was statemented, once every year we would also go to a meeting at the school with his teachers and various professionals from the local education authority. These always felt like Groundhog Day to me, as we had the exact same discussions every year. What was even more frustrating was how many times Julie and I would arrive at the school for the meeting and take our place at the table. There would be about ten name badges situated around the table, including ours and his teachers, and if we were lucky one person out of six from the local education authority would show up. Once, much to Julie's embarrassment, I refused to stay for the meeting. I was furious, as I was very busy at work and had juggled numerous appointments to make the meeting, and the so-called professionals, whose job it was to track Will's education and make sure his needs were being met, couldn't be arsed to turn up. Julie said I had come across as a grumpy bastard, and I probably did, but I preferred to think of it as passionate!

At home, we had the full Sky package so William had access to countless different channels and hundreds of films. We also had a PlayStation, which he loved to play on. Something that always surprised me was his ability to navigate around the Sky channels and particularly the PlayStation. To do it required a lot of reading, and yet he did it with ease. I'd question him on how he was able to do it, or tease him and suggest that he'd been pulling our legs all this time and he could actually read. Will would just say he didn't know how he was doing it, he just could. There were obviously some graphics that would help him, but he definitely appeared to recognise whole words. I discussed this with his teacher Duncan and he said they would try teaching him how to read by whole word recognition, and perhaps, with enough repetition, he would start to learn.

One of the joys of having access to so many films was introducing William to some of my favourites that I had grown up watching. I decided it probably wasn't a good idea to let him watch *Death Wish* or *First Blood*, but he did love all the Bond films, *Back to the Future*, *Bugsy Malone* and the old classics like *Mary Poppins*, *Bedknobs and Broomsticks* and *The Wizard of Oz*. But the ones he loved most were the Pink Panther films, which were a firm favourite of ours growing up. To me there was no greater sound to come home to than William laughing his head off. The fight scenes between Inspector Clouseau and his Chinese manservant Cato had him falling out of his chair with laughter. However, I had neglected to consider the consequence of introducing him to these films.

I came out of my bedroom one morning at about six o'clock, half-asleep in my dressing gown, and as I walked past the bathroom William jumped out from the dark behind me shouting 'Cato' at the top of his voice and launched a full-scale attack on me. I nearly had a childish accident! It became a game between us that Will loved, and for someone who couldn't shut up for a minute, he was scarily good at staying silent for ages while hiding in various places ready to jump out on me. I was a bloody nervous wreck most of the time.

Weeks could go by without an attack and one morning I walked downstairs into the lounge completely unaware that anyone else was up and awake. The lights were off and everything seemed exactly as it was when I went to bed. We have a window seat in the lounge and the curtains come down low to the floor, hiding the seat behind it. As I opened the curtains, William jumped out on me, shouting the obligatory 'Cato' as loud as he could. He scared the life out of me, and instinctively I grabbed him in mid-air, twisted my body and threw him onto the sofa. Will lay there in shock and then decided that in real life I was actually an assassin! He does have a very vivid imagination, but this was one fantasy that I didn't try too hard to dissuade him from. Obviously, his daddy was a trained killer for hire!

When you turn on the television often it will return to the last channel that was being watched, and more and more often I noticed that William had been watching what I referred to as the 'God Squad channels'. I don't mean something harmless like *Songs of Praise*, these were the 'Hallelujah, praise the Lord, you're forgiven for all your sins now send us all your money' type of programmes. William was obviously very impressionable and I'd be subjected to a long line of questions regarding his sins and going to hell. Every time I found him either watching them, or proof that he had, I threatened to stop him watching television. This went on for months, and one evening, when Darren was home again and we were sitting in the dining room catching up and enjoying a good bottle of wine, William knocked on the door and asked if he could come in as he had something really important to tell me. He was very excited.

"Dad, you know that Bible nonsense that I'm not allowed to watch, well I've found something much better than that. There are ladies in bras and they're lying on sofas holding a phone up and saying call me. Can I call them, Dad?"

As he was saying it he was mimicking the girls caressing their breasts and holding an imaginary phone to his ear. Somehow, I managed to avoid Darren's eyes and keep a straight face.

Very calmly I said, "No, absolutely not, William, you are not allowed to watch those programmes either. It costs a lot of money to make those calls and its only for adults. If I can't trust you to make good decisions, I'll have to take away the controller."

As he left the room Darren and I looked at each other with huge grins forming, but both knew we couldn't laugh out loud straight away. When Will was out of earshot Darren started to giggle and said, "Fucking A-star parenting, Mr M, how the hell did you keep a straight face? I nearly spat wine all over myself."

"Yeah, that was tough. Well, at least we know where his preferences lie now, that's one less thing for me to worry about and, luckily, he can't make phone calls," I said, and then we both started laughing.

A few weeks later William was supposed to be getting ready for school one morning but was playing in his room. Julie was getting increasingly frustrated with him as he'd been in his bedroom for ages and was going to be late for his bus. She knew he wasn't getting dressed and, at the end of her tether, she shouted loudly up the stairs, "William, come on, you're going to be late! I know your game."

Immediately we heard his door swing open, and an irate William came stomping down the stairs into the lounge looking really angry and shouted at his mum at the top of his voice, "I'm not gay!"

I said, "I'm happy to hear that, Will, but that's not what your mum said, she said she knows 'your game'. Now get dressed quickly or you'll be going to school in your dressing gown."

I don't think Julie or I had really appreciated how difficult managing this stage of Will's life would be. In many ways, he was still extremely immature, but he was having all the same feelings as any other boy about to turn fourteen, but without the ability to understand them. 'Appropriate' became the most overused word in our house. I lost count of how many times he came downstairs in loose-fitting pyjamas with an erection. The natural reaction would be to shout at him and tell him off, but we didn't want to embarrass him or make him feel that it was shameful. One day, Emily's friend Maddie was at our house and William was moaning about having sore shoulders and asked Emily if she'd massage them but she refused. Maddie obviously thought Emily was being mean, so she offered to do it, but within seconds of her rubbing his back he got an erection. Maddie looked embarrassed, and Emily screamed at him, "Oh my god! William, you are disgusting, I can't believe you sometimes!"

"It's not my fault, Emily, it just happens!" William shouted back.

We had a chat with Maddie, who was really cool about it, and then later Julie spoke to her mum, who was also very understanding. However, it was acutely embarrassing for Emily, so I had numerous chats with Will about self-control, what was appropriate, and what stuff should remain private. Fortunately, they were very easy conversations to have as he wasn't in the least bit embarrassed and was more than happy to talk openly with me about his feelings.

One day I was scrunching up some old newspaper to put on the fire when Will shouted out, "Wow, stop, Dad. Can I have this one please, for my bedwoom? Don't put it on the fire."

He was holding up a double-page centre-spread that had numerous photographs of the very pretty and voluptuous actress Helen Flanagan modelling a range of bikinis.

I smiled and said, "Yeah, okay, mate, no problem. Remember though, keep it private in your bedroom, this is just between us men, okay?"

About thirty minutes later he called down from his bedroom and asked me to come and look at what he'd done. You can imagine what was going through my mind, but he seemed desperate for me to see. I knocked on his door and waited for him to say come in. I opened the door slowly and peered in, and he was sitting on the floor, holding up the newspaper, as pleased as punch.

"I know it's pwivate, Daddy, so I won't tell Mummy or Emily, but I'm very improud of it."

The whole page had been coloured in. Helen was now yellow and red with purple boobs, and she had a moustache and a beard, and even horns in some of the photos. He was so chuffed with his artistry.

I said, "Yes, Will, I'm very impressed with your colouring in and I'm very proud of you."

I emphasised the words 'impressed' and 'proud' as I said them; but I'd done that his entire life, he still preferred improud.

When Emily got Prince we also bought her a mobile phone. Many of her friends had mobiles way before her, but I had never seen any reason whatsoever for Emily to need one. However, it was reassuring when she was out riding on her own to be able to contact us if there was a problem. William was extremely jealous and wanted his own mobile, but I was adamant it was a complete waste of money and wouldn't be persuaded.

Before their fourteenth birthdays Julie told me that she was going to get him one to make things fair, and thought that he could be trusted to use it sensibly. I didn't share her faith.

On the morning of their birthdays, William unwrapped his first present – it was a Scooby-Doo outfit and he was absolutely made up. But when he opened his other present and found a new mobile phone I'd never seen him look so excited. Julie had programmed in the important numbers he might need, and very patiently spent hours teaching him how to use it. It was a pay-as-you-go phone and Julie had put ten pounds-worth of credit on it. We both spoke to him at great lengths about using it only if he absolutely had to.

The day after his birthday was Sunday. He woke up early and from his bedroom he called his Nana Di, at about five in the morning – she told him it was very early so he hung up. He then made several other calls to the other programmed numbers, and we only realised what he was doing when Julie's phone started ringing and woke us up. He was told off and made to understand that he was wasting his credit and would have to apologise to everyone he'd called. After a long lecture he promised us faithfully that he now understood.

Julie went to work at the hotel later that morning, and after a couple of hours her mobile started ringing. It was William.

"William, you know you are not allowed to call me at work, this better be very important," she said angrily.

"Mummy, it is very important, George wants to talk to you."

His phone then died as he had used up all of his credit in one morning. Julie never did find out what our dog wanted to talk to her about!

Unfortunately, I had been proved right about the mobile, and it wasn't long before William started losing interest in his chickens, as I'd said he would. As his dad, these were the times I wanted to be proved wrong; I wanted him to show me that he was ready for these responsibilities. We found ourselves constantly having to tell him to let them out in the mornings and feed and water them. One day he wouldn't get out of bed, and Julie went to his room to get him up and he was hiding under his duvet pretending to be asleep.

Julie said, "It's no good pretending, William, you need to get up and let your chickens out. Stop being so lazy."

He threw his duvet back and shouted, "I hate those bloody chickens!"

Although we continued to make him look after them, it caused so many arguments that over time we ended up doing more and more of the work. One morning I told him he was not allowed to leave his bedroom or have any breakfast so he would understand what it was like for his chickens to be stuck in their coop. He looked at me as if I was the cruellest man in the world and then, of course, made me all the usual promises that he now understood and would look after them properly. But it didn't last. As Julie reminded me, though, we tried, and at the very least we were getting free eggs.

Ron was now eighty-nine and was suffering with two very bad knees that prevented him from doing the work that he loved. He was spending more and more time indoors and June had noticed some worrying changes in him. She took him to the doctors believing he may be suffering from dementia, which was later confirmed. June was going through some old photographs that she thought might help him to see, and she came across one of him when he joined the army, aged seventeen. She stared at it in disbelief, and then came straight over to our house to show us. She passed it to me and asked who it was in the photograph. I said it was obviously William; it was black and white, and he was dressed in a military uniform, but it was definitely my son. I thought it was brilliant and asked when she had got it done, believing it to be one of those photos where they dress you up and photograph you in black and white to create the impression it was from a bygone age. She called Julie over and asked her the same question and then William and Emily. Everyone thought it was William, including William himself. She took great delight in pausing for dramatic effect before telling us that it was actually Ron when he first joined the army.

I have never in my life seen two people who were not identical twins look so alike! It was extraordinary, and also incredibly moving. When we were given Will's diagnosis we were told he would not grow up to look like us, or indeed anyone in the family, as the extra chromosome would alter his looks. We had just accepted the word of an expert. To see indisputable evidence that in fact William looked exactly like his granddad was very emotional.

In July 2011, I turned forty, and celebrated with another really big garden party. The weather was glorious, and of the one hundred and eighty people I'd invited only six didn't make it. The adjacent field was turned into a car park with portable loos scattered around. There was a large marquee, a disco, a hog roast, and enough alcohol to put the village to sleep. There were barmaids serving behind a make-shift bar, and waitresses serving shots around the garden. One of my brother Pete's best friends is a very funny comedian, called Phil Butler, and I'd arranged for him to do a spot. He was so funny and had everyone in stitches with his hysterical routine.

I'd also booked a guy called Pete Sands, who is a brilliant Elvis impersonator. Pete was using The Retreat as his changing rooms and, in true Elvis style, the build-up was huge. Blaring out of the considerable speakers the soundtrack from '2001: A Space Odyssey' started and then, as the intro music blended into 'See See Rider' and everyone started to scream, the doors to The Retreat were opened and Elvis appeared, to rapturous applause. It took a few seconds for us all to realise the Elvis accepting everyone's adulation was, in fact, William! He was dressed in his own costume, complete with the wig, and looked magnificent. No one had any idea that he had sneaked his costume into The Retreat and obviously taken some choreography from Pete. He moved around the crowd with the energy and confidence of a seasoned performer as we all clapped to the beat of the song. He was sensational! He then took his customary bow and moved aside for the 'real' Elvis, who sang all of our favourites superbly. William was in his element and, unlike several years before at my last big party, there were no tantrums when his moment was over.

I was aware that both Darren and Steve had planned to say a few words on my behalf. I wasn't sure what I was letting myself in for, but I'm certain it wouldn't have all been complimentary! However, when Elvis had finished his set, Emily took the microphone and gave a speech about me that had everybody drying their eyes. It was beautiful, so well written and incredibly moving. The confidence she displayed to speak so well in front of that many people was extraordinary. Both Darren and Steve said there was no point in trying to follow that. I had a garden full of all my friends and family, and my two children had made me proud beyond belief. At that moment, in the areas that matter, I felt like the richest man alive.

Chapter Eighteen

I'll Sleep With My Glasses On

D uring the summer holidays of 2011, William had his first few days out with a group called Project My Time, who are a subsidiary of a Dorset-based charity, Diverse Abilities Plus. Julie had been told about them from other parents at Will's school. We had never once asked for any help or respite care for William and really had no clue as to what was available. Now he was fourteen we were worried he would get bored just hanging around the village every day. I was working full-time and Julie had just qualified to be a mobile nail technician, in addition to working part-time at the hotel, and although it was on a very small scale, and started off with just a few friends, she was keen to slowly build her business. Julie managed to get Will booked in to go out one day a week throughout the holidays, which gave her some much-needed respite. He absolutely loved it. He was always very confident meeting new people anyway, and these days out gave him a chance to meet new friends and try new experiences. During that summer holiday he went to places like Weymouth, Swanage and the New Forest, and got to try abseiling, kayaking, sailing and rock climbing. We were so happy for him, and also pretty annoyed at ourselves for having not explored these opportunities for him before. I think Julie and I had never considered that we needed help, as we had a large circle of friends and a close family, but for William's sake I really wish we'd done it years before.

When I meet other parents of children with special needs and disabilities I am always in awe of how they cope. Often their child's needs are far greater than William's, and sometimes there is only one parent to do the caring. The stress it can put on them is unimaginable and they really do deserve all the help and support they can get. I honestly never considered William to be a burden, he was our son, and we just got on with taking care of him. To be fair though, whenever friends or family members had him for the day they were always honest enough to admit they found it exhausting, albeit lots of fun. I guess you just get used to what you have to do on a daily basis and, even though Will was a teenager, we were still having to do many of the things we did for him when he was a toddler.

Towards the end of that year, and with Christmas fast approaching, we asked William what he would like from Father Christmas – Emily was right when she'd said he would still believe for a very long time! Sometimes his behaviour could be very testing, so it was nice to still have that bribe 'Father Christmas is watching' up your sleeve. We were completely taken aback when he said he wanted a double-bed. Bearing in mind that for every Christmas for the past few years all he'd wanted was dressing-up costumes, this was real progress. I explained to him that even though Father Christmas was magic, a double-bed might be a step too far to get down our chimney, but perhaps we could buy him one.

"Listen, Will, I think it's a great idea, and we'd be happy to get you one," I said. "The only problem is, your bedroom is not that big. I'm not sure that one would even fit."

He looked so disappointed and had obviously given it a lot of thought. Julie glanced in my direction and pulled a sad face, so I said, "Come on, then, Will, let's get a tape measure and we'll go and see if one will fit in your room."

"Oh my god! Fanks, Dad! I am really excited, come on, let's do it now," he said, with a huge smile.

I walked and he ran upstairs, and skipped across the hallway and very nearly bashed his head on a beam – he seemed to be getting taller every day now. When I walked into his room my first thoughts were *no way, it will never fit*, and then I remembered you can get smaller doubles that are only four feet across. I handed him one end of the tape measure and, after several failed attempts, he managed to hold it steadily against the wall.

"Right, Will, it just fits, but it's very tight and you wouldn't even be able to have your bedside table anymore," I said, with a tone and a look that should've suggested it's a nonstarter.

He glanced at his bedside table and said, "That's okay, Dad, I'll sleep with my glasses on."

It was one of those melt-your-heart moments, when all you can do is agree and say yes. In his mind, the sole purpose for his bedside table was to sit his glasses on when he went to sleep and he'd solved that problem.

Although William had proved unable to handle the responsibility of a mobile phone, I thought it was important to make sure he had a good telephone manner. Whenever I heard him talking on our landline to a friend or family member he would only give one-word answers. Sometimes he would only nod or shake his head, perhaps not understanding that the caller couldn't see what he was doing. Julie or I would often stand next to him while he was on the phone and prompt him to give more detailed responses, and remind him of the importance of being polite and asking questions, not just answering them. It had obviously felt too much like work for him and he'd started to avoid the telephone altogether. He used to jump up when the phone rang to answer it, but he'd taken our help as criticism and it had knocked his confidence. He now ignored a ringing telephone altogether, and several calls had been missed as we ran down the stairs while he just sat watching TV, refusing to get up and answer them. Eventually I decided enough was enough. I told him he was fourteen years old and he could bloody well man-up and answer the telephone when it rang.

A few days later, Julie and I had just sat down to eat our dinner in the dining room when the phone started ringing in the lounge. Julie immediately put her knife and fork down and pushed her chair back and went to get up.

"Darling, sit down, William's in the lounge, he'll get it. I've told him he's got to start answering the phone, it's bloody ridiculous," I said.

By the third ring we heard him say, "Hello . . . yes . . . that's right."

"See, I told you he'd answer it, enjoy your dinner," I said, a little too smugly.

No more than ten seconds later we heard Will say very enthusiastically, "Yes, please, I want some new windows."

"Oh, for fuck's sake," I said as I jumped up and ran to retrieve the phone from him.

Just a few days later Will almost gave me a heart attack. I was about to walk into The Retreat when he flung open the lounge window with the phone in his hand and screamed that Rachel was dying. I started sprinting back down the garden, and was nearly at the cottage when he shouted it was Reggie who was dying. Now I wasn't sure if it was my sister-in-law or her dog, but either way it was bad. When I ran into the lounge and picked up the phone, whoever was there had hung up and Will was back in his armchair watching television. Breathless and panicking, I asked him who was dying and very nonchalantly he said, "Oh, sorry, Dad, I heard her wrong. Megan is driving."

All too often William would only hear parts of a conversation or get his words completely wrong. He was sitting watching television one day, and I was in the kitchen chatting to Julie, when he shouted from the lounge, "Mum, Dad, come in here quickly, look at this, I really want to do some hardcore."

We gave each other a worried look and moved swiftly through to the lounge in case he'd been too adventurous with the Sky controller again. He was watching a programme about freerunning. The narrator was explaining how it had evolved from the original parkour.

"Dad, please, please, can I? I really want to do some hardcore," Will pleaded.

"Don't we all, son, don't we all," I said, while Julie just rolled her eyes at me.

William's habit of flicking had been progressively getting worse over the last couple of years. What started out as something he had probably just copied from a classmate had now escalated to a point where he was doing it several times a day, for long periods of time. Apparently, this is referred to as self-stimulatory behaviour, or stimming. It is described as the 'repetition of physical movements, sounds or repetitive movement of objects common in individuals with developmental disabilities'. We would find pens, pencils, cutlery and even chopsticks stuffed down the side of his armchair or bed where he could retrieve them quickly and flick while no one was looking. Every child is different, and William knew that what he was doing looked silly and was hiding it from us. I had no experience of behaviours like this, but I didn't like it. As far as I was concerned, it was just a habit he had learned and he could unlearn it just as easily. I'd get cross with him when I caught him and plead with him to stop doing it. I am sure the experts would tell me I wasn't dealing with it correctly, but I would snap whatever he was using to flick with when I caught him. It didn't seem to bother him though, as sometimes he would snap it himself and tell me he knew it was silly.

Shortly before the twins fifteenth birthdays in March 2012, I was chatting to William in the kitchen about turning fifteen and how grown up he'll be, and I asked him if he'd like me to take him out and choose some new glasses. I'd been concerned for some time that his glasses reminded me of the National Health ones that some unfortunate children had to wear when I was growing up.

"Would you like that, Will? We'll get some really cool ones. You'll look really handsome," I said.

He didn't seem too interested and was just looking out of the kitchen window.

After a while he said, "Dad, why don't we have curtains in the kitchen?"

"Talking of curtains! Blimey, Will, that's a bit random, I suppose because no one can see into our kitchen so we don't need them."

"Well, that is what I would like for my birthday," he said confidently.

"You want curtains for the kitchen? For your birthday?" I said with a smile.

"Yeah, then everyone can enjoy my birthday present."

"That's very sweet, Will, but I'm sure you can think of something you'd like more, but if that's what you want I'll talk to Mum."

"Thank you, yes, I really want curtains. Daddy, if you have enough money, can I have the pole as well?"

He really was such a kind-hearted young man. We never did get curtains, but he soon forgot about it, and I did take him out shopping and let him choose whichever glasses he wanted. Annoyingly, the ones he chose were Ray-Ban, and he looked great in them, but at two hundred pounds they were the most expensive in the shop, and he broke them within the first week. I was starting to understand why Julie had always got him the cheaper ones and was kicking myself too. I reckon the curtains would've probably cost less and certainly lasted longer!

A few weeks later, William came home from school and told us he had been chosen to be in the school choir. He was beaming with pride and spent the next few days singing all the time around the house. Shortly after, we received an invitation to attend 'Beaucroft Sings 2012', an evening of songs performed by the teachers and students for the parents. Although I would, of course, attend to support William, secretly I wasn't really looking forward to it. It was one of those things you just have to do rather than want to, but I started to feel a little more optimistic listening to Will practise every night in his room as the songs were pop songs and not the hymns I had imagined.

It was a beautiful summer's evening and we arrived at Beaucroft and took our seats in the packed school hall. The headteacher, Mr McGill, welcomed us all and explained how hard the teachers and students had been working and that we were in for a treat. He wasn't wrong. Including William there were about forty children up on stage of various ages and all with their own individual challenges. Behind us was a large screen with the words to the songs projected onto it for the students to follow. As William couldn't read, he had learned all of the songs off by heart. William and every other child on that stage sang so beautifully, and with such pride, it was without doubt one of the most moving and memorable nights of my life. Will's teachers, Duncan and Sally, sang Coldplay's 'Fix You', not an easy song to sing, but they were brilliant. The first line of the song, *'When you try your best but you don't succeed '* really struck a chord, and very nearly reduced the audience to tears. For the entire evening I listened to those beautiful children sing with a lump in my throat the size of a grapefruit, and wasn't sure if I'd be able to hold it together. At the end of the show we all gave them a standing ovation, and demanded an encore, but clearly the children had planned something a bit different. We were asked if any of us would be prepared to get up on stage and sing with them, and before the teacher had finished her sentence William was shouting from the stage, "Come on, Dad, I want you to sing with me! Please, Dad, please!"

Everyone started laughing, and most of the audience turned to look in my direction, so I had little choice but to get up and join Will. Fortunately, several other parents stood up and followed me up onto the stage. It was a very special moment. William was so proud to have his dad next to him, and although a McFly song was not in my repertoire I really enjoyed sharing that stage and singing with such amazing children. When we finished, Mr McGill stood up and addressed us again, but this time with tears in his eyes. He was so proud of his students and I remember thinking how refreshing it was for a headteacher to show such emotion.

I will never forget that evening and the profound effect it had on me. I was there to watch and support William, and I was immensely proud of him; however, William was a natural performer, who loved nothing more than being the centre of attention and entertaining people. For most of the other children it was an enormous challenge to be singing on stage, in the spotlight, in front of so many people. For each and every one of them it was a tremendous personal achievement. Some people would consider stepping into a boxing ring to be brave; but to my mind, there were forty children on that stage demonstrating what real bravery was.

Chapter Nineteen

It's Just Comedy

Although getting Emily her horse had probably helped in delaying the onset of the difficult teenage years, it was only a delay. Soon after the twins turned fifteen, Emily began to transform into an argumentative little shit. Although back then she hadn't yet found the courage to treat me disrespectfully, she was treating her mum like something she'd stepped in. I am sure that my sister must've given our mum a hard time, and mums and daughters the world over will have experienced the same, but I found it unbearable. Coming to terms with having a son with special needs was very tough to deal with, but this was a close second. The nature of my business is that when it's good, it's really good, but there were so many times when deals I had worked on for ages would fall apart and I'd earn no money for months at a time. I could be under enormous amounts of stress, and the last thing I needed was a war going on when I got home.

Whilst William was incredibly challenging he was still very sweet and always wanted to sit with us and have a cuddle. He was kind and thoughtful and very polite. Emily had always been the same but, all of a sudden, we seemed to be sharing our home with the Antichrist. It's not as if she had completely gone off the rails, she wasn't taking drugs, sleeping around or getting arrested, she was just incredibly unpleasant to live with. I have always felt that as long as my home life was good I could cope with whatever the world threw at me, but now I was coming home every evening to referee battles between my wife and daughter, and I was just no good at turning a blind eye or switching off to it. It nearly drove me insane watching the daughter I had put so much effort into raising well, become a horrible little cow. It didn't matter what I said to her, it just didn't get through. I guess some people can't cope with stress at work, money worries, health issues or the death of loved ones. I always felt I coped well with all of those things, but the constant rows at home pushed me to my limits.

I am sure what made it so hard for me to accept was that, of all people, Julie just didn't deserve it, as she was a brilliant mum to the twins. Julie is loved by everybody who knows her; she is kind, thoughtful and very caring. Between her part-time job and running her small nail business, the hours she works equal that of a full-time job. Although I do a lot to help around the house she does far more than I do and our home is always immaculate. Every single day she would spend time with her dad and help her mum with his care. And she somehow made the time to go to the gym four times a week too. Every day she gets up before six o'clock and does not stop all day, some evenings getting back from the hotel after eleven. She has an amazing amount of energy, but the most impressive thing of all, is she does everything with a smile on her face.

If finding your perfect girl is like playing the lottery, then I had hit the jackpot. Like all of us, she has her faults, but when you've loved someone for so long it's those imperfections you come to love the most. Almost daily Julie gets her words wrong. One day she told me how pleased she was to be home safely as she'd been driving erotically all day; sometimes it was so busy at the gym it was just pandemonia. She often quotes well known sayings incorrectly, too, like 'last year this time' and 'he was very thought after'; but my favourite is when she shows me her boobs because, according to her, they are really 'up and Adam'.

Listening to Julie tell a story it takes so long to reach a conclusion that she is now affectionately known as 'real-time Julie'. My friend Steve came up with the nickname as he swears her stories take the same amount of time as the experience that she is describing. Playing board games with her is hysterical. One day we were playing Who's in the Bag? with Steve and Emma. The bag is full of cards with famous people's names on, and the object of the game is to describe as many famous people as quickly as possible before the sand-timer runs out. Because she was against the clock, Julie panicked and described a hat that you have to wear on a motorbike. I quickly pointed out that we were playing who, and not what is in the bag! I turned the card over – and the answer was Hamlet. However, she has an intelligence that I admire; an ability to see things exactly as they are; to cut through all the bullshit and see things in a very logical, straightforward way. While I might over think and analyse every little detail of what someone has said or done, she sees it in a way that is so simple that it's brilliant. I have the best wife in the world, and I love my daughter unconditionally, so it was naturally heart-breaking that they were battling so often.

I often felt very guilty, because Emily had inherited my way with words and an annoying ability to argue one's case. She could tie Julie in knots and, in her immature mind, she'd believe she was right just because she was better at making her point, even though, clearly, she was in the wrong. To be fair, Emily was just like any other fifteen-year-old girl pushing the boundaries, and it was only because I cared so much that it hurt so much more. I knew that we'd brought her up well, and it was just a phase, and while you should never wish the time away, there were many times I could have happily pushed the 'fast-forward to twenty years old' button.

I was chatting to Emily one day and she said, "Dad, if science made it possible, and even if it was really expensive, would you pay to get William and me cloned?"

I said, "I'd get George cloned first, as he's my favourite, and if I had enough money left then, yes, of course I would."

"You're joking, aren't you?" she said, whilst giving me a sideways look.

I said, "Of course I am, Emily, who'd want another one of you?"

Although at this stage in her life she made things tough, it made me appreciate what an absolute pleasure living with William was. For all of the obvious daily challenges we faced raising William, in many ways, at this age, it was far easier. He didn't want to stay up late at night, he wasn't on social media with all the related problems, and there were no exams to get stressed over. Whatever clothes we bought him he'd wear and would be really grateful, and he wasn't in the least bit bothered by brand. He didn't answer back, let alone argue. Some boys his age would be getting into trouble, getting drunk, doing drugs or getting a girl pregnant. We had none of those worries with Will. He talked incessantly, and needed assistance with almost every aspect of day-to-day life, but he was an absolute pleasure to spend time with. Of course, there were many difficulties, some of which I couldn't have anticipated.

William loved a cuddle, and being so innocent he saw nothing wrong in shouting from his bedroom, "Dad, can we have a cuddle? Can you get on my bed for a special cuddle?"

In Will's mind that would just be a really nice cuddle, and there is nothing wrong in a dad giving his son a hug, but William had no comprehension that his choice of words might sound concerning. Then I'd be faced with a dilemma: I could say nothing and hope that he stopped referring to it as 'special'; or I could try to explain to him that the expression 'a special cuddle' conjures up all sorts of disturbing images in people's minds, the problem being, if I did try to explain to him he would tell me he understood, then the very next person he saw he would tell them that his dad doesn't want him to talk about special cuddles. Damned if I do; damned if I don't!

One Saturday morning I was rushing to get out of the door. I had been selected to captain the Remedy Oak golf team in an away match against Camberley Heath. It was an hour's drive and I wanted to make sure I was there early and was running a little late. I got all of my gear together, and shouted my goodbyes, but when I got into my car I realised I had forgotten the team sheet. As I ran back into the house I heard William shout from the shower, "Mum, I need you to clean my helmet."

"Okay, I'll come and do it in a minute," Julie shouted back.

It stopped me completely in my tracks. I thought, *what the hell goes on when I'm not here*?

It took me a few seconds to remember they were doing a sponsored bike ride that morning. His innocence was lovely, but the older and bigger he got, the more challenging it was to deal with.

William absolutely loved Halloween night. He needed no reason to dress up in any outfit he fancied, but an occasion where everyone dressed up was heaven to him. All of the children in the village meet up at a designated cottage, and two or three of the mums go with them around the village trick-or-treating. Afterwards, they go back to the village hall to share out all of the sweets and have a party. Many of the cottages put scary Halloween decorations up and it's a great night for the children. It didn't bother William one bit that he was the oldest and biggest amongst them. Before he left the house, I asked him to tell me what it was he had to say when someone opened their door.

With great pride he said, "Cock all treat."

"No, mate, that's definitely not what you say," I said, whilst trying not to laugh.

"Yes, it is, Daddy! It's cock-all-treating," he said, with absolute certainty.

I used the five minutes we had before he left to explain to him in great detail why it was most definitely trick-or-treat and not cock-all-treat. He promised me that he understood, and as soon as he left I asked Julie how long they'd be gone, and if she wanted to play his version of the game! She reminded me that Emily was upstairs in her room so, unfortunately, we weren't allowed to play!

My cousins Jack, Sam, Harvey and Finnian were by now all pursuing their own careers, and understandably were following in their parents' footsteps. Their mum had found fame as a dancer and their dad, Tony, was an accomplished actor, before becoming a successful businessman. Jack and Sam had both attended drama college – Jack had an obvious talent for acting, whilst Sam, who could also act, was a fantastic singer. My godson Finnian was now a successful model and, after a being a very talented trampolinist, Harvey landed a job with the world-renowned Cirque du Soleil. It was his dream job and his first role was in the 'Michael Jackson Immortal World Tour'.

Towards the end of 2012, the tour was coming to London and all of the family had tickets to go and see him at the O2 Arena. I was not sure I'd ever seen William more excited. The show was an electrifying mix of death-defying stunts, singers and dancers, all performing in front of huge screens to Michael Jackson's songs, with the man himself coming to life as a giant hologram. Harvey had one of the most dangerous jobs in the show as a high-flyer, swinging around on trapezes and bungee cords at the highest point of the arena; it was spectacular. I am not sure that William blinked for the entire show. For the following few weeks the only music blaring from his room was Michael Jackson's and, to be honest, I've never been a fan so it was a painful few weeks!

One Sunday lunch we'd just sat down at the dining table. We had friends round, and as we were about to start Will put his knife and fork down and said, "Excuse me, everyone, I would like to say grace."

We all exchanged a few funny looks before Julie said, "We never do that, Will, but you can if you really want to."

We all put our cutlery down, and as Will bowed his head, put his hands together and closed his eyes, we all took his lead and followed him.

Very slowly and deliberately he said, "Dear God, I hate Michael Jackson because he died, and my dad is a big fairy. Amen."

We all started laughing and I said, "Well, thanks for that, Will. I love you too, mate."

"It's just comedy, Dad, and now you may all start your lunch," he said with a smile.

It was very typical of William to come out with something random and funny, but I realised during lunch that this was different from before. I watched the mood around the table change and he'd deliberately used comedy to improve it. He had obviously decided that we were all a bit quiet so he said something funny and we all started having a great time. All his life he'd been a funny boy. When he was really young it might have just been a funny, well-timed look; then as he got older it would've been something he did that just happened to be funny. Now he was saying things to deliberately make us laugh.

A week later we were sitting in the lounge watching the annual *BBC Children in Need* television programme. I guess, like most households up and down the country, there comes a moment in the show where what you are watching tugs so hard at your heartstrings that you can't just sit back and do nothing. For us it normally follows the same pattern: Julie starts crying and then gives me a look, which I understand to mean 'get your bank card out'. William would normally start cross-examining his mum then on why she was crying, but this time he didn't, he quietly and respectfully let her cry. Then the show took a more light-hearted turn and they showed footage of Pudsey Bear visiting various children around the country. William watched for a while and then, without looking away from the TV, he said, "Dad, why doesn't Pudsey Bear come and visit me?"

"Because you're not a child in need are you, mate," I said dismissively.

He pulled a funny face and said, "Der! I think you're forgetting I've got learning problems!"

I was noticing such a change in William – and his humour was just one aspect of it. He was growing up, maturing and developing into a lovely young man. I spoke to Julie and told her it was time I explained to him about Father Christmas. As Christmas was just over a month away she was really reluctant to let me do it, but I said I was adamant. He was fifteen and I was sure he was mature enough to keep the secret from little children, and it was important for his development to know what is and isn't possible. I gave my speech a lot of thought before calling him downstairs from his room for a chat.

"William, I have something very important I want to talk to you about. It's about Father Christmas. There is a secret that mums and dads keep from their children. It's a wonderful secret that brings lots of happiness. Now you are a young man I can tell you, but it is very important that you then keep that secret."

"Okay, Dad, you can tell me," he said in a very serious tone while nodding his head.

"All these years when you've believed that Father Christmas had brought you your presents, it was actually me. Father Christmas is pretend; it's a lovely story that brings children a magical feeling at Christmas, but it's just that, a story. I put your presents there. Do you understand, Will?"

He was certain I was teasing him so I gave him the same speech, several times, in many different ways, until he assured me he understood. As he got up to leave he turned to me and put his index finger to his mouth and said very quietly, "Don't worry, Dad, I won't tell Emily."

I went into the kitchen and told Julie how well it had gone, that he wasn't upset, and that he completely understood now. Ten minutes later Julie and I were sitting in the lounge and he came downstairs again.

"So, Dad, you are actually Father Christmas and you can vanish like that?" he said, and simultaneously clicked both his fingers.

Julie started laughing and said, "Yeah, he's got it completely, Rich, nice work."

It did take me a few more efforts to finally get Will to understand, but he took it very well. We talked about the impossibilities of one man delivering presents all around the world at the same time. I showed him all the places in the world on a globe, and we joked about a fat guy trying to get down our chimney. I also told him he still had to be well behaved if he wanted a nice Christmas present. That was when he told me he wanted a drum kit. He'd been having lessons at school, and with his natural rhythm he was doing really well and he loved it. Fortunately, we had The Retreat, and with a bit of furniture rearranging it would fit and he could make as much noise as he wanted in there.

I said, "Will, I think a drum kit is an excellent idea, but let me look into it first, I think they cost a lot of money and I'm not sure I can afford it."

"Yes, you can, Dad, just get a Payday loan," he replied, and gave me a big theatrical wink.

I laughed out loud and said, "You have definitely been watching far too much television!"

"It's just comedy, Dad, just comedy," he said, with a smile.

After a couple of weeks of researching various drum kits, I had just about given up on the idea. They were far more money than I would ever spend on the children at Christmas and I told Julie that we'd have to think of something else. An hour or so later I got a phone call from a guy I had done some business with in the past – he was hoping I could find him a house to buy as a refurbishment project – and we got chatting about what he was doing these days, and he told me he owned a music shop but had moved away from the retail side and now focussed mainly on teaching music.

"I don't suppose you've got a drum kit sitting around looking for a home? My son has been having lessons and he's desperate for one for Christmas," I asked.

"You're in luck, Rich, I've just finished clearing the last of the gear out of the shop and only yesterday I put a drum kit into storage in my garage at home. It's been used, mainly for teaching and a few gigs. Give me a drink and it's yours."

Two days before Christmas I drove over to Bournemouth and collected it and put it together in The Retreat while Will was out. On Christmas Day morning we were sitting around the Christmas tree unwrapping our presents and we handed William his; it was about the size of a shoe box and he looked a little confused. A few days before, I had seen one of those miniature toy drum kits that you might put on your desk, for sale in a charity shop window. I thought it would be fun to wrap it up and pretend that was his present, to see his reaction. He unwrapped it and stared at it for a few seconds before jumping up and cuddling us both and telling us he loved it. Julie shot me a glance and mouthed, "Bless him."

"I'm so glad you like it, Will, and I'm sorry we couldn't afford a proper one, but I'm sure it will sound great in The Retreat, the acoustics are really good in there. Shall we go and try it now?"

We walked up the garden with Will holding his drum kit in one hand.

He said, "I know it's small, but I do like it, Dad, and like you say, I should be grateful for whatever I get."

"That's right, son, I'm proud of you for being so understanding."

I opened the door to The Retreat and said, "What do you think of your real present, Will?"

"Oh my god, oh my god, I can't believe it! Is this really mine?" he screamed.

"Yes, Will, it's yours, I was only teasing you. Go on, then. Show me how good you are."

Will rearranged the drum kit slightly, as I'd not set it up correctly, and then he started playing. He was really good, far better than I thought he'd be, and he put some music on and played for over an hour. Eventually he came back to the house with a smile from ear-to-ear. He waited until we were out of earshot of the girls and then whispered to me, "Dad, I knew you were teasing me. You really are Father Christmas, aren't you."

Chapter Twenty

Bang! And The Dirt Is Gone

I was walking George through Chettle woods one morning in early March 2013; it was a beautiful day and the promise of spring was all around. I was thinking about work and mentally visualising my appointment diary for the day ahead, when it occurred to me that it was only five days until the twins turned sixteen. It then struck me that it was exactly five days before my sixteenth birthday when I completed my last 'O' level exam and walked out of the school gates for the final time. I was transported back to that sixteen-year-old me and naturally found myself making comparisons between Will and me at the same age, the truth being there really was no comparison.

I was very mature for a sixteen-year-old, probably far too sensible for my own good, focused, driven and incredibly headstrong. I had my life mapped out ahead of me in my mind, and was determined to do whatever it took to be a success. William never thought like that; he lived his life in the moment and the idea of visualising his future was an alien concept to him. For the first time in years I was starting to fear for Will. At his age I was ready to go to work, and could've lived independently, but it was difficult to imagine a time when Will would ever be ready for that. For several weeks after Will turned sixteen every time I thought about him I would worry.

About a month or so later I was chatting to a friend, who was experiencing a really challenging time in his life. He was in debt, he believed his marriage was in trouble, and he hated his job. He was really stressed and was struggling to see a way through. I listened to all his problems, and then I gave him the best piece of advice I'd ever been given. I told him that there are only two things in this life that you are in control of: your thoughts and your actions. It doesn't matter what is going on in your life, you and you alone can decide how you think about it and what you do. Thoughts are powerful things, and in any given moment you can change the way you think, and the moment you take action things will change.

As I was saying the words I realised that somewhere along the line I had forgotten this life-changing advice myself. I had been concentrating on all that William didn't have or couldn't do. I could continue to focus on all that was missing, or decide to change my thinking in that moment. I made a conscious decision to be mindful of all the joy that William brought to everyone he met, and to focus on every one of his qualities and strengths. I thought about Julie and me, and every challenge we had faced together raising William, and realised that he was actually the glue in our family, it was Will that had made us so strong. I thought about that sensible, driven, headstrong sixteen-year-old, and although there is no doubt life experience would've naturally altered me, it was William's influence that'd had the greatest impact on who I was today.

There is huge debate over nature verses nurture when it comes to raising children. I was most definitely in the nurture camp, and always believed that it was purely down to good parenting. But time and experience had altered my perception of this. In my friend Steve's career as a criminal lawyer, he had encountered numerous examples of people that he referred to as the 'bad seed'. These individuals had carried out despicable crimes, and yet the family they'd come from had never had a parking ticket between them. His experience convinced him that people are just born the way they are. More often these days I am minded to agree with him, but I still want to believe good parenting makes a difference. We have a responsibility to do the very best we can to raise our children to be decent human beings, but I guess we have to accept that ultimately the die is cast at conception. We can be the best sculptors in the world, but if the rock is poor we are doomed to fail.

When I think about the early studies of boys with XYY, and particularly how a higher percentage than normal end up in prison, I wonder if any of those individuals had been diagnosed at a young age. With correct, early diagnosis, surely their future would've been brighter? If William had not been understood, shown love or been taught right from wrong, I am convinced he would be locked up by now. He is so impressionable, and if the correct values had never been drummed into him I am certain he would've turned out very differently. There will always be differing opinions with the nature-nurture argument, but personally I like to believe that the two probably play an equal part.

Julie and I had both assumed that William would continue his education in the sixth form; or as is referred to at Beaucroft, Post Sixteen. It was a shock when we discovered that this wasn't guaranteed and we would have to apply for a place. We also had to explore other opportunities that were available to him, visit local colleges and make a case for why we believed his education would still be best met at his current school. We made appointments and visited Bournemouth & Poole College and then Kingston Maurward in Dorchester. I found it really frustrating having to take the time out to make these visits, as it felt like such a waste of time. Julie and I both knew there was no way Will would cope in these environments, but we still had to go through the motions. There was a possibility that Kingston Maurward might be suitable, as they specialised in land and agriculture, and we thought Will would enjoy the farming side of it. Although we both very much liked the college, the students were expected to manage their own timetables, and had the freedom to wander in and out of the college grounds. There was no way William was ready for that level of independence.

As was becoming the norm, there was countless form-filling, and much time spent keeping our fingers crossed, but eventually Will was granted a place in Post Sixteen. The really good news was Beaucroft were about to build a totally self-contained unit for the older students, and Will could continue his education there for another three years, not the expected two. It was a huge relief for us to know that he would remain where he was happy and for the next three years he would have stability.

In April the four of us went on holiday to El Gouna in Egypt. I had never considered it before as a holiday destination, but we were only going for a week and wanted guaranteed sunshine and a relatively short flight. Emily was already talking about holidays with her friends the following year to places like Magaluf and Malia, so we were sure this would be our last ever family holiday. I booked two adjoining rooms in a five-star hotel, and was particularly pleased that the hotel's policy was no guests under the age of sixteen: peace and quiet around the pool. It was only after I'd booked it I realised I was being selfish and I was worried that Will would be bored with no one to play with.

The first morning, we were relaxing around the pool when the music started blaring and the animation team arrived in a sea of colour, singing and dancing and doing their best to get everyone in the holiday spirit. I remember lying there thinking *for fuck's sake, I've booked a five-star hotel not a bloody holiday camp!* From the looks on most people's faces around the pool I wasn't the only one. William was incredibly excited, though, and immediately got off his sun lounger and ran up to join them, despite me trying to stop him. The crew were doing a well-practised dance routine that wasn't having the desired effect on us lazy sunbathers, but the atmosphere changed completely when Will joined in. He was in his element, and didn't care one bit that he didn't know the song or the correct moves. He was so funny, and started calling everyone around the pool to get up, join in, and have a good time.

For the rest of the week Will became part of the animation team. They took him under their wing and Julie, Emily and I were able to relax, switch off and soak up the sun. Will spent every day going around encouraging people to get involved in activities, straightening sun loungers and getting people clean towels. Each day he joined the team for the customary poolside dance – it was a complicated routine, but he kept getting better. Time after time we were approached by guests who just wanted to tell us that he had made their holiday and what a lovely young man he was. On the final day, he walked out to the pool with the crew, dressed in matching colourful clothes, and did the whole choreographed dance routine without putting a foot wrong. Every single guest around the pool got off their sun loungers to give him a round of applause. William was allowed to keep the clothes, and they gave him a CD with all their music on it to bring home. After a month of being back at home we all knew those songs very, very well!

On Sunday 16th June, Emily knocked on our bedroom door, came in and put my coffee down, and leaned down for a hug, gave me a kiss, and wished me a happy Father's Day. She gave me my favourite bottle of wine in a gift bag, and a card with the most beautiful hand-written words inside. She told me the wine was from both of them, but apparently Will wanted to give me something else too.

Julie shouted out, "William, are you coming in? Emily says you've got something for Daddy?"

"I have, but he's got to come into my bedroom!" he shouted back.

I reluctantly got out of bed, slipped my dressing gown on, and walked across the hallway and into his room. Will was still lying in bed under his duvet.

"Morning, mate, apparently you've got something for me?"

"I have, but you've got to come really close, Daddy," he whispered, as if it was some big secret.

As I bent down he whipped his duvet off, spun his legs around, punched me straight in the stomach and shouted, "Bang! And the dirt is gone!" and burst into hysterics.

"Thanks for that, Will, that was a good shot," I said, and left his room cursing Barry Scott and his bloody Cillit Bang adverts.

It was very much our kind of humour. I'm not sure when it started, but for years, whenever Will was daydreaming and off guard, I would walk past and give him a very gentle slap around the face and say, 'Daddy-slap'; it was just one of those silly father-son things. Whenever Will tried to do it to me, my reactions were too quick, and I'd always catch his hand in mid-air. I was quite proud of him for managing to catch me off guard for once!

Both the twins were due to finish school for the summer holidays around the same time in late June, about a month earlier than usual, as most of the country's sixteen-year-olds would have just finished their GCSEs. We were extremely relieved when Emily's were over, as she always got so stressed with exams. At her prom night she and three of her friends were chauffeured into the school grounds in a convoy of four Mini Coopers, while the music from the film *The Italian Job* played loudly from huge speakers in the car park. It was very cool, and Emily and her friends looked stunning in their prom dresses.

Beaucroft were also having a prom night, and the school had booked a small nightclub in Weymouth. The invitation said, 'dress to impress'. William was so excited, as he'd never been to a nightclub, and I was sure that he'd have plans to wear one of his funny costumes. We were very surprised when he announced that he actually wanted to wear a suit. Julie suggested it should be me who took him shopping, but I was expecting all sorts of dramas. Will had his own very peculiar sense of fashion, and I could imagine him picking out weird and wonderful clothes and me having to keep saying no and disappointing him. It turned out to be one of the easiest shopping experiences of my life. Will was tall and slim and a size small man's suit, straight off the peg, looked like it had been tailored for him. We selected a shirt and tie and he paraded around Burtons like a model, checking himself in every mirror and asking every customer he saw to confirm that he looked very smart.

Riding on the tide of success, I decided to brave it and take him for a haircut. Salons have been the cause of much embarrassment over the years – the hairdressers never knew what they were letting themselves in for when they engaged Will in small talk. He would talk non-stop for the duration of his haircut, and some of the things he'd say would have me squirming in my seat. He once asked a hairdresser if she knew that he used to be a sperm. He's told others that his dad was an assassin, and I'd buried Henry in the garden. I've heard him say his mummy gets drunk, I fart, he likes sleeping in his sister's bed, and when his daddy is not there George gets on the bed with mummy. However, this day he never said a single embarrassing thing. When we left I thanked him for being so good and told him how proud I was of him.

Will turned to look at me, smiled and said, "It's because I'm a grown-up now, Dad, I'm going to a nightclub."

I suggested we should go to a restaurant for dinner on the way home, as a nice finish to our boy's day out. Sometimes William still ate at a snail's pace and could ruin a meal out, but he surprised me again. Not only did he choose to go for a curry, which was a first, he ate about twice the amount I did, and finished before me!

At the end of the meal I said, "Will, I've really enjoyed today, you've been so well behaved and such great company."

"Are you impressed with me?"

"Blimey, Will! You said impressed and not improud, I think that's the first time ever. I am very impressed!"

"I'm grown-up now, like you. I've got a suit and I've had a curry and I'm going to a nightclub and I can have sex with sexy ladies," he replied, and pretended to fondle an imaginary pair of boobs.

"Don't ruin it, William," I said sternly.

"Sorry, Dad," he replied instantly.

On the evening of his prom Julie and I both went to his school to watch him and all his friends get on the coach. The girls all had beautiful prom dresses, and most of the boys were in smart suits. Going to a disco or a nightclub at their age was something most of us took for granted, but it was a big thing for them and the excitement was at fever pitch. Will was getting a little too animated, so I took him to one side and told him to calm down and suggested we should go and thank Duncan and Sally for everything they had done for him over the past three years. As I was shaking Duncan's hand and telling him how grateful we were, William shouted, "Mr Russell, this is a daddy-slap," and pulled his hand back as far as it would go and slapped me really hard across the face.

For a few seconds no one said a word, and I was feeling a mixture of shock and acute embarrassment, and was worried that his teacher might actually believe I ever slapped my son that hard. Then the awkward silence was broken as Duncan burst into laughter. There was nothing I could do but laugh it off; it's not as if I wasn't used to him embarrassing me in public! Will was just over-excited, and he knew he'd over-stepped the mark, but at least it did the trick of calming him down. Fortunately, the prom was a huge success. Will really enjoyed his first nightclub experience. He danced all night, and when we went back to meet the coach at the end of the night he was fast asleep in his seat.

It was going to be a very long summer break for William, so Julie had planned ahead and organised for him to go out with Project My Time on as many activity days as possible. His first day out was to Longleat, the wildlife and safari park near Warminster in Wiltshire. I had to pick him up from the coach station in Ringwood at six o'clock. He got in the car with a large bag of Haribo sweets and started stuffing them in his mouth.

"Slowdown, Will, you'll make yourself ill. Did you have a good time? What did you get up to today?" I asked.

"Umm, just stuff," he said dismissively.

"Wow, that's fascinating, mate. Come on, leave your sweets and talk to me. I want to know what you did and all the animals you saw."

He gave a big sigh and said, "Umm, seahorses."

I thought about it for a while, and then said, "Seahorses? Are you sure?"

"Yes, I'm sure!" he said confidently.

"Oh okay, they were in a fish tank, then?"

"No, in a river!" he snapped, obviously getting frustrated at my silly line of questioning.

It took me the time to manoeuvre out of the car park space before I realised what he meant. "Will, do you mean sea lions?"

"Oh, yeah," he said disinterestedly, and stuffed another sweet in his mouth.

Will really enjoyed his days out but, luckily, he was just as happy spending time in the village. There was a particularly warm spell in July, and on one of the hottest days of the year I decided to leave the office early and head home to spend some time with him. As I got to our door he opened it before I could and stood in front of me with a serious look on his face. He was wearing large, brightly coloured checked trousers, a matching bow tie, a T-shirt, over-sized shoes, a red nose and a huge colourful wig. I looked him up and down and said, "You alright, Will? Is there any reason why you're dressed as a clown?"

He screwed his face up and said, "Der! I got too hot as Scooby-Doo!" and pushed past me, shaking his head as he went.

"Sorry, mate. Stupid question, I guess," I said as he walked away, his clown shoes making a slapping sound on the patio as he went.

Chapter Twenty-One

I Don't Want To Go To Wales!
I Want To Go To Atlantis!

Despite exhaustive efforts by us and everyone involved in his education, William has never learnt to read. Although it obviously impacts on so many areas of his life, it's amazing what you get used to. When he is handed a menu in a restaurant he takes it and then waits for us to read him the choices. We still point out which is the shampoo and which one is the conditioner. When we watch the television, I read out loud any written words, like subtitles and the captions, that sometimes appear. It must be very confusing trying to follow a plot if you can't read on the screen 'One year earlier' or 'Ten years later'. I came home from work one evening, towards the end of the summer, and William was sitting in his favourite rocking chair in front of the television and a film was just about to start.

"Hi, Dad, I've just put a film on, is that okay? Can you watch it with me, please?" he begged.

"What is it? What's it called?" I asked as I lowered myself onto the sofa.

He smiled and said, "Dunno, but it says it's got violence, scenes of a sexual nature and flashing lights, and I like all of those."

As far as television is concerned, it isn't just the written word he struggles with. When we are watching the TV, it is obvious to us the difference between a drama and a documentary. We know what is live and pre-recorded, and whether somebody is acting or presenting. We instantly realise what is filmed in a studio, outside on set, or is actually CGI. Will doesn't have a clue, and often I'll have to

189

spend a long time explaining to him what he is watching. He would tell me he understood and then say something which would only serve to prove that he absolutely didn't!

After completing drama college, my cousin Jack had spent several years pursuing his dream of becoming a successful actor. Like so many in his profession he didn't get an early break and attended every audition he could. He performed in some small theatre productions, and had a few television appearances, most notably in *House of Anubis*. When the work wasn't there he would wait tables, or hand out leaflets on the streets of London to get by. He had come very close to giving up on his dream of making it as an actor when he landed his first major role at the age of twenty-seven. The BBC had commissioned a prime-time Saturday night TV series called *Atlantis*, a fantasy adventure inspired by Greek mythology, very much in the vein of *Jason and the Argonauts*. They had assembled a fantastic cast including Mark Addy, Robert Emms, Aiysha Hart and Sarah Parish. Jack was given the leading role of Jason, which was a huge break for a relatively unknown actor, and the whole family were incredibly proud of him. The first episode was due for release on Saturday evening, 28th September 2013, on BBC1. We were all really looking forward to watching it and I was sure that seeing Jack act on television would help William's understanding enormously.

Jack phoned me five days before the first episode aired and asked if I could get Will the following day off school. He told me they were expecting to film dramatic fight scenes that would be included later in the series, and if I took Will to the studio in Wales he could spend the day watching the filming and meet the cast. It was exactly the kind of magical stuff I had been fortunate enough to experience when I was young, and I was so happy for William. He had a new teacher in Post Sixteen called Sally Norman and I was a little embarrassed that my first real contact with her was asking if Will could take a day off school, just two weeks into the new term; but when I explained the opportunity that Will had been given, Sally agreed it would be an amazing experience for him and allowed him the day off.

As soon as Will got home from school I explained what we were going to do the following day. He was ridiculously excited, so much so that I started to worry about his behaviour on set and hoped I wasn't making a dreadful mistake. I talked to him for over an hour about what the inside of the studio might look like, with the dramatic sets and actors, directors and make-up artists all milling around. We spoke about the importance of being very quiet when they were filming, at which point he asked me if he could be in the show. This gave rise to another hour of talking, and eventually he promised me that he did understand.

"Right, Will, get a really good night's sleep, we've got a long day ahead of us and it's a long drive to Wales," I said as I kissed him on his forehead.

"I don't want to go to Wales! I want to go to Atlantis!" he shouted.

"Good night, Will," I replied, far too exhausted to argue.

We set off the following morning with the directions Jack had given me to get to the studio. It occupied a building that was previously a Tesco distribution centre on an industrial estate just the other side of the Severn bridge. It would take about ninety minutes to get there from Chettle. I talked non-stop for the first hour and reiterated everything I had said the night before. I also explained to Will, in great length, that although the scenes were being filmed today, it would be many months before they would be included in episodes of *Atlantis* and we'd be able to watch them on television. Will seemed equally as confused as he had the night before, but eventually he seemed to get it so I decided to take a break from talking and put the radio on. I selected the auto-tune button and on came Radio 2, and the first voice I heard was Graham Norton's – and he was introducing Jack Donnelly! It was a repeat of an interview that had been recorded the previous Saturday morning with all the stars of *Atlantis*. As I was trying to calculate the odds of turning on the radio at that exact moment, William recognised Jack's voice and immediately started waving at the radio and shouting 'Hello, Jack!' at the top of his voice! I had reached the point where I could explain no more. I spent a few minutes in quiet frustration, before giving in to the fact that it was probably far more fun in Will's world and maybe he just didn't need to understand how everything worked.

We were met by a security man, who was expecting us, and taken through the vast building to where Jack was filming. We only had to wait a few minutes before Jack had a break and was able to give us a tour of the studio. There was no need to have worried about Will's behaviour, he was transfixed by the amazing sets and spent the day in an almost hypnotic state. Each time the director shouted 'Action!' Will would grab my hand and nod to signify he knew he had to be quiet, and as soon as he heard 'Cut!' he gave the actors a round of applause. Jack introduced him to everyone on set and gave Will a day he'll never forget.

Mark Addy was really nice to Will and had a very funny chat with him.

"Who are you then?" asked William as he looked Mark up and down.

"My name is Hercules, I am the strongest man in Atlantis," Mark replied, and gave me a wink.

"Huh, I bet you're not as strong as my daddy," said Will in a very self-assured way.

Mark fixed his gaze and said, "Listen, William, no one is as strong as your dad."

Will wagged his finger at Mark. "And just you remember that," he warned.

Mark roared with laughter and said, "I won't, William, I promise."

On Saturday night we watched the first episode together as a family; it was fantastic entertainment and William took great delight in explaining to his mum and his sister that Jack wasn't really in Atlantis.

If I'd thought that one day in a studio would solve all of the mysteries of television for Will, I was very much mistaken. Knowing him as well as I do, there are still plenty of times when even I can't work out how his mind works. Some months later I came home from work and, after chatting with Julie in the kitchen, I asked her where William was.

"He went to watch a film, but I think he turned it off about ten minutes ago, he must be upstairs," she said.

I walked into the lounge and he was sitting in his rocking chair watching a film in silence.

"Blimey, mate, it's so quiet, why is the volume turned down? I really can't hear it at all, you must have excellent hearing," I said.

"What?" he said.

I smiled and repeated myself, "You must have really good ears, it's really quiet. I can't hear it at all."

"Neither can I," he said, without looking around.

"So why don't you turn it up, then?" I asked.

He turned to face me and said, "They were annoying me, Dad, so I shushed them. You know, like when I'm annoying you, you tell me to shush. I've done it to them."

"You could always just turn over, mate," I said, just in case he hadn't considered that option.

"Don't turn over, I'm enjoying it. It gets better!" he pleaded.

"You've seen it before, then?"

"Yes, I only shush that bit," he said, and looked back at the TV and turned the volume up.

On Sunday 3rd November I was driving home from the golf club in a terrible mood. I'd had a totally shit week. One of those that you just can't wait to see the back of. Every one of the property deals I'd been working on had gone sour, and I'd spent most evenings sitting around candles and throwing half-cooked dinner into the bin due to constant power cuts. For two months I'd been building a bonfire pile for the village fireworks night – it was over thirty-feet high – and after a month's-worth of rain had fallen in the week, it had become a soaking wet mound of crap. I had no idea how I was going to get that lit in two days' time. The one thing I'd been looking forward to all week was playing golf in the competition. I was playing really well, and was two under par through eight holes, when the heavens opened again and they closed the course. I was soaked through and really pissed off, and all I wanted to do was grab a bottle of wine and hide in The Retreat for the remainder of the afternoon, drowning my sorrows.

I started to feel a little better as I turned off the main road and headed towards Chettle. The rain had finally stopped and the sun had decided to show its face. I'd already slowed my speed before I passed the sign that says, 'Please drive slowly, free-range children', and I drove around the pond and turned right at the conker tree towards the village shop. I then passed the old red phone box, and pulled in by the stables on my left to let John go by in his tractor – and wondered what he was laughing about. From there I could see up the road beyond the hotel to our cottage, and it wouldn't be long before I'd have my face buried in a large glass of wine. My eyesight is good, but it took me a few moments to adjust to the vision I saw a couple of hundred yards up ahead. Strolling down the road towards me was Big Bird from Sesame Street. It was about six-foot tall and was bright yellow with funny googly eyes. I grabbed my phone and managed to take a photo and put my window down to have a chat.

"You okay, mate? I love the outfit," I said.

But Big Bird didn't slow down, it just strolled past my car, nodded its head and said, "Alright, Dad."

I drove the remaining hundred yards laughing to myself and thinking *I bet there aren't any other sixteen-year-old lads out there who get dressed as Big Bird just to go for a walk on a Sunday afternoon.* Julie told me he had been given the costume that day by a friend in the village. Will had put me in a much better mood before I'd even opened the bottle and taken my first sip! (I've learned from experience that wine tastes so much better when you're smiling!)

Later that evening, and with a belly full of roast lamb, we were sitting in the lounge in front of the fire watching television. I was making good progress on a second bottle of wine, and was trying to engage Will in conversation – never easy when he's watching a film.

"So, are you ready for school tomorrow, Willy?" I asked.

Will sat bolt upright in his chair and turned to face me with a look of rage on his face. "I am not Willy, that's not my name. I am not a willy!" he shouted at me.

"Yes, it is. You're Willy, that's your name, it's short for William," I teased.

"No, it is not, you boing-boing head! My name is William, not Willy!" he screamed, even louder this time.

I laughed out loud, not just because my teasing was having such an effect, but it had been many years since he'd last called me a boing-boing head.

"Don't tease him, Rich, you know he doesn't like it," said Julie.

"Alright, mate, sorry, but Willy is just another name for William. We call you Will, but you could be Willy, Bill or Billy. They are all just other names for William. If it makes you feel any better, did you know that the shortened version of Richard is Dick?"

"What?" he said as his eyes widened and he started to smile. "Your name is Dick?"

"Yes, or it could be."

He considered this for a moment, and then shouted, "So we are both penises!" and fell into hysterics.

By eight o'clock Will was starting to drop off in his chair so I told him it was bedtime. He got out of his chair really slowly, as if he was a very old man, stretched his arms out wide and did a huge loud yawn, farted, apologised, and then took a few slow steps towards the stairs. He then stopped, and seemed to be thinking of what he wanted to say. Then he turned towards me with a triumphant look on his face and said, "Goodnight, cock," and shut the door behind him, laughing as he went.

On Sunday 1st December I flew to Antalya in Turkey for a week's golfing holiday with seven of my friends. I have been on many lads' golfing trips over the years, and usually so much alcohol is consumed the golf can become secondary to the drinking. Although the hotel in Turkey was all-inclusive, I was determined to take it easier than normal, enjoy my golf, and get some much-needed rest. Over the past five years my business partner and I had taken on an ever-increasing workload, and I was constantly juggling my finances to keep every property deal going. We were doing well, and had really turned things around together, but the more stress I was under at work, the harder it was to cope with Will every day. I got to Turkey and, apart from a few phone calls home, I left my mobile in the safe and relaxed, rested and recharged my battery.

I got home very late the following Sunday night and was back in the office by eight-thirty the next morning. William made me a coffee and, after a quick chat about Turkey, he dropped the bombshell: he wanted to split up the partnership. It wasn't quite the welcome home I was expecting! We talked all morning and all I'll say is sometimes people can really disappoint you. To use a boxing analogy, everyone gets knocked down, it's what you do when you get back up that matters.

That afternoon I phoned my friend Spencer, who had an empty small cob cottage in the grounds of his property, and I asked him if I could rent it as my office. I was very grateful when he said yes and offered to help me move all of my office furniture. Before the week was over, I had set up and registered a new company and moved into the office. I'd had business cards printed, computer and phone lines installed, contacted every person I had ever sold a property to, and all the investors I had ever borrowed from. I had also called over three hundred branches of estate agents that I dealt with and given them all my new contact details. It's amazing what you can achieve when you absolutely have to. As the saying goes, 'diamonds are made under pressure'! It was one of the busiest weeks of my life, and could've been extremely stressful, but I'd dealt with far harder things raising my son. It certainly helped to keep everything in perspective.

Over the years, whenever I have told someone I have twins, the first question they always ask is are they girls or boys, to which I reply, 'one of each'. I'd like a pound for every time I've then been asked if they're identical! Genetic impossibilities aside, the truth is that apart from the first two years it has never felt like we had twins. And now it felt like the gulf between them had never been so great. Emily was doing two B-Tech courses in the sixth form, one in business studies and the other a triple sports diploma. She was studying for hours, working part-time in the hotel, looking after Prince and, in whatever free time was left, she'd get picked up by friends in cars to go to parties. William was like the character Tom Hanks played in the film *Big*, a child in a man's body who only ever wanted to have fun. Increasingly though, he was beginning to notice the differences, and found it really unfair that he didn't have his own laptop, mobile phone, job and friends with cars. We probably spent far too much time trying to explain why, and not enough trying to come up with a solution for him. But eventually we did.

Our friend Malcolm from the village worked in Chettle timber yard and also delivered logs to all the surrounding villages. Every weekend you could hear his chainsaw going in the woods and we asked him if Will could help out. Malcolm loved Will, and was very patient with him, and although it was only for a few hours over the weekend, slowly he became less of a hindrance and more helpful. Will loved it, he got a few pounds for his efforts, and felt like a man. For Christmas we bought him a set of walkie-talkies; it was an inspired idea. He wasn't ready for another mobile, but this way we could keep in contact with him wherever he was in the village. They worked really well, until Will started pretending he couldn't hear his mum.

"William, tea's ready, can you come home now?" Julie would say into her transceiver.

After a few minutes she'd repeat herself, and then again and again until he responded.

"What, Mum? I can't hear you!" would come his reply.

"Yes, you can! Tea is ready, come home now," she'd say, getting increasingly annoyed.

More time would pass until, "What, Mum? I can't understand you."

We would have a giggle between ourselves at his cheekiness, and then I'd take the transceiver from Julie.

"William, it's Dad, come home now!" I'd say as seriously as I could.

"Okay, Dad. Sorry, Dad," he'd reply instantly, and be home before we knew it.

We also got him an iPod that he could access the internet on, and instead of having to type into a search engine he could speak to Siri and request what he wanted to look at. Will loved it, and took great delight in telling me that his mate Cyril was much cleverer than I was as he knew everything! Although Will's speech had improved dramatically, sometimes he was lazy with his mouth and would mumble his words. He'd also get really cross with Cyril when he couldn't understand him. We've heard some of the funniest interactions between our son and Apple's intelligent personal assistant, usually about Will's fascination with anything that inflates, like Violet Beauregarde from *Willy Wonka and the Chocolate Factory*.

"Violet Bordigard," Will mumbled.

"Sorry, I couldn't find anything like that," Siri replied.

"Violet Bordigard," Will repeated.

"Hmm, I'm not finding anything for that," said Siri.

"Are you stupid?" Will shouted really loudly.

"I strive to do my best," said Siri.

"Right, I'm getting my mum on you, she's gonna sort you out!" Will shouted as he stomped down the stairs.

Julie and I went to parents' evening at Post Sixteen and it was the first time I had properly met his new teacher Sally, I liked her straight away. To do her job requires kindness, and enormous patience, but clearly she was also a no-nonsense kind of lady. As I listened to her talk about William, it was obvious that she was very fond of him and had worked him out in a few short months.

Sally said something during that meeting that I have never forgotten.

"William has very high self-esteem, which is terrific, but he also has very unrealistic expectations. Our intention is to manage those expectations without damaging his self-esteem. In Post Sixteen we are starting to look at career choices so, for example, William told me today he wants to be a policeman. What we do is say, okay that's great, then encourage him to find out all the skills that a policeman requires to carry out his role. Then he can decide for himself whether or not he possesses those and if it's realistic for him."

In that moment I realised where I'd been going wrong: William did have very unrealistic expectations; he saw no reason why he couldn't be a racing car driver today and an astronaut tomorrow. If he hit one straight golf shot he'd be 'turning pro', and if he poured his milk into his cereal bowl without spilling it, he was going to be chef. I have always just told him the reasons why he won't be able to do those things, and I always said it kindly, but ever since that meeting I have adopted Sally's method and now I help William to work it out for himself. It's never too late to learn, and I knew she had inadvertently shown me a way I could be a better father.

Chapter Twenty-Two

See Dad, I Told You I'd Be Famous

In early January 2014, William walked into our bedroom one morning and very confidently announced that he was going to do a skydive. At least once a day he would come up with some new thing he wanted to do or be, but this seemed different. I'm not sure whether he'd seen it on television, or if he'd remembered that I had done a skydive with Finnian a few years before, but he was adamant he wanted to jump out of a plane. I was really surprised; he'd never shown any tendency before to being an adrenaline junkie, and wasn't exactly comfortable with heights. He asked me loads of questions about what it was like, and the more I talked about my experience the more excited he got. However, I was convinced he'd change his mind the next day; but he didn't, he really was deadly serious.

I found the website for the company with whom I had previously jumped and explained to Will that a tandem skydive from fifteen thousand feet would cost three hundred pounds. All over their website were testimonials from people who had jumped for various charities. The idea was that they raised money through sponsorship to fund their jump, and what was left over went to their chosen charity. We talked about this as an idea for him and he said he wanted to do it for Diverse Abilities Plus. I told him I thought that was a brilliant choice. Then he really surprised me. He said he wanted to pay for it himself so Diverse would get all the money. I thought this was incredible, for although he has very little understanding of money he certainly hates to part with his!

I said, "I think that's very kind of you, Will, but three hundred pounds is a lot of money, you'll have to use all of your Christmas money that you have left over. Then you'll have to ask everyone for money on your birthday and it will all go towards paying for the skydive. You won't get any presents."

He nodded his head and said, "I know, Dad, I don't mind, I want to say thank you for all my nice days out."

I was really moved. It was a lovely moment, and a wonderful gesture, but I wasn't going to start telling the world just yet. I told him I thought it was best to do it in the summer, and I knew that before then, there was still every chance he would change his mind about jumping out of an aeroplane.

As time went on William was still very enthusiastic, but Julie and I were worried that he might completely freeze when it was his turn to jump. When he's scared, his body goes completely rigid, and we could only imagine the dramas he might create when the doors were opened or, worse still, when his feet were dangling out of the plane at fifteen thousand feet. Julie said she thought I should do it too, so that I could be there in case he freaked out.

"I've done one with Finn," I said. "No, you should do it, you'll love it. You've done a bungee jump before, you'll be fine, it's the same only much higher. I'll pay for you to do it," I said, with a big grin on my face.

Julie looked instantly worried. "Oh, but darling, you're not scared. You love all that crazy stuff. I don't think I could do it, I'm nervous just thinking about it. I think a little bit of wee has just come out."

I laughed out loud and resigned myself to the fact that it would be me going up in the plane with Will. However, several nights later, Julie had drunk a few glasses of wine and was talking to Will about his skydive. Fuelled with Dutch courage she told him if he wanted her to, she'd do it with him. He was ecstatic, and started jumping up and down and clapping his hands – and that was that, there was no going back for her!

Two months later, on 12th March, Will and Emily turned seventeen. William opened his cards and happily handed over all the money he'd been given without any complaint.

We had paid for some driving lessons for Emily, but a few weeks before she had snapped two ligaments in her ankle tripping over a step. I felt so sorry for her, as she had to wear an orthopaedic boot, and it was going to be a long time before she could start learning to drive. I wouldn't have blamed her if she'd been really upset, but she remained very positive and focussed on the fact that she'd now have longer to save for a better car. I had always told Emily that she would have to pay for her own car and insurance. I had to when I was her age, and it had made me really appreciate and take care of my first car. The truth was, I was always going to help her out, I just didn't want her to know it, so she'd save her money. As far as she was concerned, the only thing I was going to contribute were the two-pound coins I had started collecting in a jar.

For three years Emily had worked part-time in The Castleman and had saved half of everything she had earned. She wanted to work more, but the hotel couldn't give her any extra hours so she got another job working in the village shop. On her first day, I went in to buy a bottle of wine, and as she wasn't eighteen she had to ask the manageress's permission to serve me. The wine was eight pounds and I handed her a twenty-pound note. She rung it into the till, paused for just a moment, and then smiled as she handed me my change – six two-pound coins. I never said a word, I just returned her smile and walked out of the shop, thinking *what a smart cookie!*

William was also in the wars. On Easter Sunday, about six weeks after his birthday, he was trying to ride his bike without his hands on the handlebars. The younger boys in the village were doing it successfully, but Will lost his balance and hit his head on a wall. He had a big bump and a nasty-looking cut that was bleeding profusely, but he tried to play it down as he knew he should've been wearing his helmet. However, it looked serious enough to warrant a visit to Salisbury A&E.

About thirty minutes later we were sitting in the hospital; it was packed, and we knew we were in for a long wait. Not the Easter Sunday we'd imagined. I was killing time reading a magazine, when Will grabbed my hand. He had a worried look on his face and motioned for me to look up. There was a large group of guys walking noisily through the hospital doors; they were all wearing biker's leathers and any visible skin was heavily tattooed. As they walked past us I recognised the patch on their backs identifying them as part of a local Hells Angels chapter. Everything about them seemed wrong, and I was sure they were intent on causing trouble. Julie caught my eye; she knew I'd already be working out which one I'd hit first if it kicked off, and I understood her look was a silent plea to not get involved. They stopped in the middle of the waiting area, had a quick chat between themselves, and then in unison shouted out loud, "Okay, kids, we're the Easter Bunnies, who wants an Easter Egg?"

I hadn't even noticed the bags they were all carrying. They each produced loads of Easter eggs and started handing them out to all the children. It was such a kind thing to do and a wonderful thing to witness . . . and a perfect example of why you should never judge a book by its cover. William was most put out that they ignored him and didn't give him an egg. The fact that he was seventeen and nearly six-foot tall was completely lost on him. Eventually, Will's name was called, the cut on his head was glued together, and we were asked to keep an eye on him in case of a mild concussion. Usually Will would drive us mad whinging about an injury, but he never mentioned it, all we heard for the rest of the day was how unfair it was that he hadn't been given an Easter egg!

Although Will was still very immature, there had been a marked improvement in him since he joined Post Sixteen. He was generally calmer and seemed to demand a lot less of our attention. Consequently, Julie and I would often forget he was in the next room and he was quickly becoming a terrible eavesdropper. I say terrible, not just because it's rude to eavesdrop, but because he was really bad at it! After we'd finished talking, Will would start interrogating us on all the parts he'd missed! It didn't matter how many times we told him it was rude to listen in to other people's conversations, if he could hear it, he felt he was included. I was the same as a child, but smart enough not to let on that I'd been listening; whereas Will couldn't keep anything to himself.

Knowing that he was bound to be listening, and even more certain to repeat what he'd heard, Julie and I started spelling out certain words in conversations so he couldn't follow it all. But even if we were talking freely in front of him he would inevitably misunderstand the conversation. I was watching the news one morning in the lounge and there was a feature on the growing problem of depression and mental illness. Julie was in the kitchen and I shouted out to her, "Julie, I can't believe what I've just heard, it's really shocking. Apparently for young men in this country, suicide is the most common cause of death."

Will sat bolt upright in his chair with a look of horror on his face and shouted, "I'm not gonna catch that, am I?"

I took Will out shopping one day and we stopped on the way home to get the car cleaned at one of those handwash places that keep cropping up everywhere. When it was finished, the smiling Polish manager approached me and said, "There you go, sir, is that better for you? Nine pounds, please."

William said, "I'll give you ten."

I handed the guy ten pounds, and he thanked me and walked off.

I turned to Will and said, "Listen, mate, it's not up to you if I give them a tip, they haven't actually done a very good job!"

Will said, "Oops, sorry, Daddy. I was scoring him."

Once again, William had misinterpreted what was being said, but the laugh we had about it all the way home in the car was worth far more than a pound of my money.

Julie and I count ourselves extremely lucky that we have always had family and friends who have been willing to help us out and look after Will when we've needed a break. A night away or a weekend to stay with Steve and Emma has made such a difference for us over the years. In June 2014, we had our first holiday on our own together for twelve years. My mum and dad had Will to stay with them, and Emily had the cottage to herself for the first time ever. I told her if she wanted to see eighteen she'd better not have any parties. I had booked us a week in a beautiful hotel in old town Corfu, and there was absolutely no comparison to our experience twelve years before in the tatty apartment block in Cephalonia. Everything was so much better, except my poor attempts at Greek, they were still pathetic!

We were lying on our sun loungers around the pool on the second day, talking about how unbelievably relaxing it was without having to worry about William, when simultaneously we both realised that this was how it would be from now on. The twins were seventeen, and they had been on some amazing holidays with us over the years, but now it was our time again.

Every summer Chettle has a village fete and it was undoubtedly one of Will's favourite days of the year. During the time that we lived in the village, it had grown and evolved into something that now closely resembles a festival. Susan's daughter Alice runs a very successful events company in London, and she took on the fete as her baby and grew it spectacularly. Hundreds of people come to enjoy everything from your standard cake stalls, wellie-throwing, dog shows and tug-of-war, to the rather unusual cow-pat-bingo, pimp your puppies, and a 'Miss Chettle Contest' where none of the contestants are female! In the evening there is live music, and most people party until they drop. Every penny of profit goes to charity – and these days that can be several thousand pounds. On the day of the fete, William will go to the field about nine in the morning to help set up and will not return home until around midnight, when he's exhausted from dancing. The only time he will pop home will be when he wants to change into another one of his costumes, sometimes several times during the day.

In the week preceding the fete I had lots of long conversations with Will about not wasting his money on junk. I told him he could try his hand at all the stalls and buy whatever food and drink he fancied, but I didn't want him spending the money we'd give him on stuff that he didn't need. Over the course of the week, we must've spoken for hours about this and he promised me faithfully that he would be sensible. There was part of me thinking it was only one day and so what if he bought a load of rubbish, but I'd been trying for so long to get him to understand the value of money. In the past, at previous fetes, I'd seen my money leave his pocket faster than John Wayne can draw a gun!

Every year I have donated some of my old clothes to sell on the clothes stall, and that year I was able to have a huge clear out. I'd got back into training and lost a lot of weight, and everything was hanging off me. Early on the morning of the fete, Will helped me carry a few sacks of clothes up to the field, and I left him there with ten pounds in his pocket and instructions to make it last as long as he could. I then headed off to the golf course to play in the club championships, which unfortunately had fallen on the same day. My handicap was now down to three, and I was one of the favourites to win. Annoyingly, I played like an idiot, and came back to the fete several hours later not in the best of moods. I walked around until I found Julie and the first thing she said was, "I take it you gave William ten pounds to spend?"

"Yeah, but with distinct instructions not to waste it on stuff. Why?"

"Try not to be too cross with him, darling, but he spent it all on a leather jacket . . . the trouble is, I think it was yours!" she said, and pointed towards him as he was approaching.

It was a really hot sunny day and Will was walking awkwardly towards me in my old thick black leather coat, holding his arms out straight so the XXL size jacket didn't fall off his small shoulders. I had a complete sense of humour bypass. I'd played golf like a donkey, wasted all week trying to teach Will the value of money, and someone had sold my very expensive leather coat to my own son for a tenner! I'm not sure what I was madder about, the fact that Will had wasted my money yet again, or that someone on the clothes stall had undersold my coat so considerably! I composed myself enough to explain to Will that the reason I'd given it away was because it was too big for me, he was half my width, and it looked ridiculous on him. He promised me he'd try and get his money back and headed off on his mission. The next time I saw him was about an hour later, by which time I'd had a word with myself and cheered up. He was stood next to the cider tent holding a pint and sporting an enormous pair of oversized rubber shoes and wearing a pair of flying goggles over his eyes. He looked at me, smiled and shouted, "Look, Daddy, look what I've bought. Have I made you happy now?" and put his thumb up.

I laughed out loud and said, "Yes, mate, that's much better, very wise purchases."

Many years before, when the twins were about eleven, I joined Facebook as it was the easiest way to keep in touch with Darren in whatever hell-hole he was working. He'd moved around a lot since Kabul, but none of the places would've ever featured on *Wish You Were Here*! I had previously been very negative about Facebook, but before I knew it my list of 'friends' had grown and I was back in regular contact with old school friends and people I knew from around the world.

For a while my posts were the usual holiday photos, and boring stories about a particularly good round of golf, which would inevitably lead to a load of banter and abuse from my mates. But one day I wrote a post about something funny Will had done, and I was inundated with likes, comments and private messages telling me how much it had brightened their day. I started to post photos of Will walking around Chettle in his various costumes, and share the funny things he said and did – and each post about him got an incredible response. I always showed them to Will, and every time he asked me if he was now famous. I always said no, not yet, Will, but maybe one day. I've had numerous phone calls from friends telling me they were having a really tough day, but seeing Will on Facebook had put such a big smile on their face. I've also been stopped in the street by people I don't know, who have been shown my posts by a mutual friend and just wanted to tell me what a special boy my son is.

A month before Will was due to do his skydive I posted a status about it and shared a link to his 'Just Giving' page, hoping a few of my friends might be kind enough to sponsor him. I know from my own experience how often I am asked to sponsor someone, so I wasn't expecting too many people to bother. I couldn't believe the response. Every day the figure kept rising, and each evening I'd show Will his charity page and tell him how much he'd now raised for

Diverse Abilities Plus. I read him all of the wonderful comments people had posted, and I had never seen him look so proud. I have some wealthy friends, who were kind enough to sponsor him fifty pounds, but it was the five-pound donations from people I knew were struggling financially that really touched my heart. Unfortunately, due to the weather, Will and Julie's skydive had to be postponed – twice. Will found the disappointment very difficult to cope with, but any delay was welcomed by Julie. Finally, a third date was arranged for Sunday 31st August.

I woke early on the day and opened the curtains. The sun was shining and there wasn't a breath of wind! I woke Will up to tell him the good news, and he was ridiculously excited; Julie, on the other hand, looked so nervous I thought she might throw up.

After a light breakfast we got in the car and headed off to the skydive centre, which was just the other side of Salisbury. Julie was really quiet in the car, and quite obviously very scared, so being the loving, sweet husband that I am I started to wind her up. I talked about parachutes not opening, and told her to make sure the straps were tight enough as they could come loose and she'd fall away from her instructor in mid-air. The angrier she got with me, the more Will laughed. She told us we were both horrible and turned the radio on to drown us out. I couldn't believe our luck! Gary Barlow's song 'Let Me Go' was playing. As it got to the chorus, Will and I started singing along to the lyrics at the top of our voices: '*Fly high and let me go!*' Thankfully, Julie saw the funny side of it and started to relax a little.

After the initial registration and training there was a couple of hours to wait for their slot. Loads of our family and friends turned up to watch and support us, so we had plenty of fun while we waited. Finally, it was their turn, and we all wished them good luck and waved them off as they walked across the field to board the plane. Julie looked as white as a sheet; whereas Will seemed to take it all in his stride. I'm not the sort to worry about what might or could go wrong, I was just hoping that Will would not freak out and they both remembered to keep their eyes open and enjoy the incredible views of Salisbury Plain and Stonehenge.

It takes quite a long time for a small plane to reach fifteen thousand feet, but eventually we were able to spot what looked like several tiny dots appear through the clouds. It was the first time I had felt any nerves at all. I didn't let on, but I was desperate to see their parachutes open, and all I wanted was for my wife and son to be back on the ground, safe and in my arms. After several minutes we watched William land safely, followed very shortly by Julie, and as soon as she was unstrapped from her instructor she ran across the field to Will and they threw their arms around each other. It was incredibly emotional to watch. They were both on such a high and the smiles said it all: they'd both loved it! They walked out of the landing zone and back behind the safety fence and everyone was cheering and clapping them and giving Will high-fives. I gave them both a hug and told them how proud I was.

Julie said, "I loved it, Rich, it was amazing, but there was no need at all for me to do it. Will was so calm, I think he was the most chilled one in the plane."

Will was euphoric and said, "I just want to do it again, Dad, can I do it again?"

The atmosphere was electric, and Will didn't stop talking all the way home, he was buzzing. When we got home I opened the champagne and did a final count up of how much William had raised. I had hoped that he might get a few hundred pounds, but he'd raised a staggering two thousand two hundred and seventy-five pounds and, because of his generosity, every penny was going to Diverse Abilities Plus! A week later, we went to their offices in Poole and presented them with a cheque, and Will was featured in their magazine. That month he was their number one, star fund raiser. *The Bournemouth Echo* did a double-page spread on the story, and I read every word of the article to Will. He was beaming with pride and put his arms around me, kissed me on the cheek, and said, "See, Dad, I told you I'd be famous."

Chapter Twenty-Three

I Love You Hundreds

The one thing any parent will tell you is how quickly time seems to pass you by. The first driving lesson I gave Emily was in Julie's car on the off-road tracks around Chettle in October 2014, when her ankle had finally healed. As I switched seats with her and she got behind the wheel I had a flashback to that moment outside the maternity ward when I was struggling to belt the twins into their car seats for the first time. Where had seventeen and a half years gone? Miraculously, we managed to get through her first lesson without one raised voice, and she was surprisingly good for a first attempt.

Emily had managed to save two thousand five hundred pounds to buy and insure her first car. I was really impressed, and after she had completed a few proper driving lessons and passed her theory test I set about finding her a car. I still have contacts in the motor trade and was able to find her a really good deal on a new shape Vauxhall Corsa that was on her list of favourite cars. The car cost more than she had, but I put the rest towards it and paid for her first year's insurance. She was over the moon. I did attach two conditions though: she had to take her brother out often, and pick me up from the golf club when I'd had a drink!

Although time can pass us by, I am sure that we can all agree that ten minutes is just that, ten minutes. Or one-sixth of an hour, or six-hundred seconds. Julie and I have learned to accept that there are three notable exceptions to this rule: when I promise that I'll be leaving the golf club in ten minutes, Julie understands that means at some point in the next thirty minutes, in exactly the same way I know how long I'll be waiting when Julie or Emily tell me they need ten more minutes to finish getting ready – which is the second exception. The third exception is Will's ten minutes. So far, I have not been able to accurately calculate how long that is. It could be anything from a minute to never! I use all sorts of made-up units of time to try and help him. One day we needed to leave the house in ten minutes, so I told Will that is the same amount of time it takes to play two songs on a CD. After ten minutes had gone and I was waiting at the door I then heard really loud music start playing in his bedroom. Frustrated, I ran upstairs and found him dancing around his room, playing the Kazoo and wearing nothing but his pants!

"Will, what the hell are you doing, mate? We are supposed to be leaving now!" I shouted over the noise of his stereo and the world's worst-sounding instrument.

He looked at me as if I'd gone mad and shouted, "But you said I had time to play two songs!"

Will has never understood time and it remains a magical mystery to him. He begged us to buy him a watch for Christmas. I did my best to help him understand that it was a waste of money as he couldn't tell the time, but he just looked at me as if I was dumb and said, "Umm, der! The watch tells the time."

Although Will's logic was somewhat confused, we gave in and bought him a digital watch with a big screen and large, easy-to-read numbers. On Christmas Day, and for several days after, Will gave us a running commentary on the time. It was like having a speaking clock walking around the house. He would proudly update us as each minute passed.

"Seven dots four one. Seven dots four two. Seven dots four three," he would announce, with great pride, even though it meant nothing to him.

Early in February 2015, William came home from school looking as pleased as punch and told us he had a girlfriend and her name was Daniella. She was in the year below Will and had joined Post Sixteen at Beaucroft in September, at the start of the term. Julie told me she had seen her with Will at school and she was a really lovely girl. Daniella has Down's syndrome and had previously always been taught in a mainstream school. Will told us they were in love and were going to get married and live together in their own house. It was very sweet, and they started to make video calls to each other in the evenings after school. Daniella was definitely the sensible one in the relationship, and we'd often hear her telling Will to calm down and not be silly. Whenever they said their goodbyes you'd always hear them say to each other, 'I love you hundreds'.

Julie bought a Valentine's card for Will to give to Daniella – she was always so thoughtful like that. I walked into the dining room that evening and Julie was asking Will what he wanted to write in the card, the idea being that she would then write it down on a piece of paper and he could copy it into the card.

He said, "Can you put 'I love you very much, be mine forever'. Also, 'I want to take you for a Chinese meal but you'll have to pay'."

I laughed out loud and said I thought it was perfect, but Julie insisted he came up with a more suitable comment. She then very patiently sat with him for what seemed like half the evening as he painstakingly copied each letter of the sentence into the card.

On 12th March 2015, the twins turned eighteen, two days after Julie had turned the dreaded forty. Whilst Julie was doing her best to forget her age and wanted her birthday to pass relatively quietly, we wanted to celebrate the occasion for the twins. Our local pub is The Museum, which is in the village of Farnham, just a mile from Chettle. It's a beautiful country pub that has become rather popular with celebrities since Guy Ritchie and Madonna bought a property close by, several years ago. We invited our families and loads of friends, and the pub did us proud with an incredible buffet. Will very proudly produced his passport as proof of his age, and the staff kindly invited him behind the bar so that he could pull his own pint. It was a fantastic night, but the highlight was when my family wheeled in Will's present: they had all chipped in and bought him an electric scooter. Although Will was not in the least bit jealous that his twin sister had her own car, having a scooter with an engine made him feel just as grown up. He looked like all his dreams had just come true.

Eight days after their birthday, Emily passed her driving test on her first attempt, and we started to see a lot less of her. Now she had her own transport our cottage became little more than a free hotel to her, a place where she slept and ate some meals. I can't blame her though; I know I was the same as soon as I got my first car.

Turning eighteen had quite an effect on Will, but not one I was expecting. For a few days he developed a really bad attitude and I heard him regularly answering his mum back. I picked him up on it and told him that I wasn't going to put up with his behaviour. I couldn't believe his response. He looked me straight in the eye, shrugged his shoulders and said, "Dad, I'm an adult now and I can do what I like."

I bit my lip and told him he was right, he was an adult now, and with that status came new responsibilities. That day I made him hoover the house, get the logs in, make all the beds, empty the dishwasher, walk George, tidy his room, dust the house and clean the bathrooms. He went to bed that night tired and fed up, and when he woke up the next day he came into our bedroom, pulled his most angelic smile, and said, "Dad, if it's alright with you, I really don't want to be an adult anymore."

I remember thinking *you and me both, son.* Thankfully, it had worked and he instantly reverted to being the sweet and polite young man that he is.

Before the end of that school term we were advised by Will's teacher to start looking at his options for when he left Beaucroft, even though that was still over a year away. Sally was aware that we'd never had a social worker for William, despite Julie making several requests to social services over the years. Apparently, we had never met the criteria, whatever that means! Sally told us that it was now vital that Will had a social worker, as all too often young adults with special needs can fall off the radar when they leave school. A social worker would be able to help us secure the funding for a college placement for Will and, heaven forbid, if something happened to both of us, at least he'd be known to Social Services. As hard as Julie had tried in the past, now we couldn't afford to take no for an answer. In these situations, it's the squeaky wheel that gets the oil, so we were advised to make as much noise as we could to get Will what he needed.

After several months we were finally successful. Will was assigned his own social worker, and a really lovely lady came to our house one afternoon to meet him and assess his needs. She spent four hours with us filling in forms, while being treated to what Will called his 'amazing fashion show'. Whenever he wasn't needed to answer any questions he went upstairs and came back down wearing a different costume. She met Mr Blobby, Big Bird, Scooby-Doo, Willy Wonka, a Power Ranger and the Honey Monster, to name just a few. I imagine it's one meeting that she will never forget. She left us with instructions to start visiting various colleges, and took her mountain of paperwork with her. That was the one and only time we met her. Sadly, just a few weeks after our meeting, she went on long-term sick leave and never returned to her job. After several further months of chasing, we were told they couldn't find her paperwork and we'd have to go through the whole process again.

Emily finished school, and soon after we found out that she'd passed both her B-Tech modules with very good grades. She managed to get herself an apprenticeship in events management, which was what she wanted to do and something I was sure she'd have a natural talent for. We were really very proud of her.

Julie and I visited loads of the local colleges and explored every opportunity for William but couldn't find anything suitable. We then got really excited at the prospect of Will attending a college for performing arts, as he had always been such an entertainer. I did some research on the internet and found a residential college called Orpheus that was for people just like Will. The only problem was it was in Surrey.

We made an appointment and set off one morning on a journey that was in excess of one hundred miles. We were full of optimism, and really excited to think we'd found the perfect place for him. Two hours later, and with the M3 at a standstill, we had to give in and turn around. We were so disappointed, but by the time we arrived home we'd made a decision: Will wasn't ready for a residential placement, and neither of us were ready for him to move out. Will was initially upset, but soon decided that performing on stage was something he'd like to do now and again and not as a career. Once again, we were back at square one.

It was a really stressful time, as obviously Will's future was at stake and, as busy as Julie and I both were, we had to make the time for all of these visits. We couldn't even begin to imagine what Will would do if he left school without something in place. Ironically, we eventually found a college that we felt would best serve his needs that was only thirteen miles from our home. Julie, Will and I visited The Sheiling School together, and we all fell in love with it. It was in a beautiful country setting and Will looked really at home there. It offered the flexibility for students to attend each day, and if and when they were ready they could stay residentially. We felt that we'd finally found the perfect place for Will to continue his education. We filled in an application form and, just a week later, we had a call from a new social worker called Simon and we fixed an appointment for him to come and meet Will.

Simon initially cheered us up no end when he told us the original paperwork had been found and we wouldn't need to spend another four hours filling out the same forms. He spent a long time chatting and getting to know Will, and we told him about all the colleges we'd visited and that we'd just applied for a place at Sheiling. I'd been warned to expect a battle to get the funding, so when he told us he didn't think it was right for Will I thought this was his way of turning us down. After all our time and effort, he seemed to be dismissing it without even a consideration for my son's future. I hit the roof. Julie looked incredibly embarrassed, but I didn't care, I was at the end of my tether and he was going to get both barrels. Normally when I raise my voice people start running for cover but, to his enormous credit, he was calm and composed.

He politely let me finish my rant and then said, "Mr Matthews, I totally understand your frustrations, and I can see how passionate you are about your son. My point is this, do you believe that further education will be of any benefit to William? With the greatest of respect to all of his schools, he's never mastered even the core subjects, and I suspect he never will. I'm just suggesting that a work placement might better serve his needs."

I was quiet for a few seconds as I allowed his words to sink in, and then it felt like somebody had just let the air out of my tyres. He was absolutely right. There was probably nothing whatsoever to gain for Will in any further education, we had just never considered that there were any other options. If we could find Will the right working environment he could learn skills that would be of real benefit to him. We were back at square one, again, but at least this time, Simon had put us on the right path.

Up until just a few years before I'd always assumed that Will would live at home with us forever. It was just one of those things I'd accepted. He was our son and we loved him, and for as long as he needed us to take care of him we'd be happy to do it. Through meeting other parents in similar situations, I realised that isn't always for the best. There were assisted living homes where Will would be able to have some level of independence, while still having his needs cared for. If there came a time when Will was ready and wanted to move out, then I would support him completely, but all the talk of residential colleges had made me realise just how much I'd miss him at home.

At his worst, he can make me want to scream in frustration. He talks incessantly about nothing, and demands an answer to every one of his random questions. He obsesses about every new thing he has, and makes really daft decisions on a daily basis. He can embarrass me terribly in public, and everything has to be explained to him ten times in ten different ways. I hate how strict I've had to be with him, and there have been so many times when I've really struggled to cope and thought it was all just so unfair.

At his best, he is one of the kindest people I've ever known. He is innocence personified and wants nothing more than to make people smile. He loves to fantasise and sees the world as the truly wonderful and magical place that it is. He reminds me how to have fun, to find humour in everything, and to show kindness to everyone. He tells me he loves me every single day, and always wants a cuddle. He has an amazing sense of humour, and no one has ever made me laugh as much as Will does.

In December 2015, we were sitting in the lounge watching an episode of *The X Factor*, and Julie and I were enjoying a bottle or two of red wine. One of the contestants sang her song and, after she'd finished, Julie leaned forward, pointed at the TV and said, "She was bloody brilliant!"

Will turned in his chair, somewhat shocked, and said, "Mummy, don't swear."

I said, "Don't be so ridiculous, William, that's hardly swearing, is it."

His eyes widened in excitement and he said, "Can I say a swear word, then?"

"If you feel you really have to," I said nonchalantly.

"Can I say the F-word? Please, Dad?" he pleaded.

I glanced at Julie for her approval and said, "Go on, then. Just once, though."

Will leaned forward in his chair, pointed at the TV and shouted, "Bitch!"

We laughed so much and, ever since, bitch has always been the F-word in our house.

A few weeks later, at the beginning of January 2016, William was sitting in his chair watching a film. I was upstairs when I heard him start shouting really loudly.

"Hello, hello, hello! Who's there?"

I came downstairs to see what was going on, but William was now just staring at the TV again.

"Why were you shouting, Will?"

He turned to look at me and said, "Oh, I thought I heard the doorbell."

It took a few seconds for his words to sink in before I said, "Will, we haven't got a doorbell."

"Oh."

"In fact, we've never had a doorbell."

"Oh."

"Besides, if we did have one you couldn't just sit on your lazy arse shouting hello, you'd have to go to the door and answer it."

He just smiled, shrugged his shoulders and said, "I'm glad we haven't got one, then."

Time was marching on and the pressure was building to find Will the perfect place for when he left school. Emily went off to work every day now, and it hadn't escaped Will's notice how hard it all seemed. He was very apprehensive about going to work, which only made us doubt the decision we'd made. We had another meeting with Simon to voice our concerns, but he brought along some information on a couple of local community farms. High Mead Farm was near Longham, just the other side of Wimborne, and it was described as a 'therapeutic farm offering a range of activities for those with learning and physical disabilities'. Holtwood Community Farm was closer to us, and it was a more traditional farm, but was also run for people just like Will. Simon was confident that he could build a strong case to get the funding for Will to attend one of these farms five days a week. They both looked amazing, and when we showed them to Will he got really excited. He'd grown up in the country and loved animals, tractors, being outdoors and working with his hands. For the first time Julie and I could visualise a future for our son when he left school.

The three of us visited Holtwood and then High Mead, and we all thought they were both amazing places. It was suggested by each of the farms that Will spent a day there to see if he fitted in and would be happy. He did just that, and loved his time at both farms. The trouble was, he just couldn't make up his mind which one he preferred. Julie called Simon and told him how much Will had enjoyed his day at both farms and asked if there was any way he would be allowed to split his working week up, two days at one and three at another. We were thrilled when Simon said he thought it might be possible. We filled out all the application forms and kept everything crossed for what we were warned could be a long wait.

For the last few months at Beaucroft, William and his friends in Post Sixteen were attempting to achieve the Bronze Level Duke of Edinburgh Award. Julie and I were both aware it was a huge challenge for Will, but whenever we asked him what tasks he had to complete he would close up. With a glint in his eye he would just touch the side of his nose and say, "You'll have to wait and see at my leaver's day."

He had never kept a bloody secret in his life! It was intriguing, but I fought the urge to push him further as Will was clearly enjoying the suspense. Julie and I knew he had to complete a long walk with overnight camping, but that was about the extent of our knowledge.

Will's last ever day at school was Friday 24th June 2016. Just eleven days before, and after a battle that had lasted for nearly eighteen months, I got a phone call from Simon. He told me that he was delighted to inform me that the funding had all been agreed. Will would be able to attend Holtwood Community Farm Monday to Wednesday, and High Mead Farm on Thursday and Friday. Transport was also being put in place for Will to get there and back each day. All we had to do was give him a start date. If Simon had told me face to face I would have picked him up and hugged him. The relief was immense.

On the 24th, Julie, my mum and I arrived at Beaucroft to watch the leaver's ceremony, and we filed into the Post Sixteen building with all the other parents, friends and families. We had also taken Sandra with us, who had been Will's escort on the bus for the past few years. She was already tearful and told us that she was considering retiring, as she just couldn't imagine working another day without Will on her bus. Sadly, June was unable to attend as Ron now required constant care at home. She was one lady who truly believed her vow of 'in sickness and in health'.

The students were all sitting at the front wearing Duke of Edinburgh hoodies. Mr McGill addressed us first; he was clearly very emotional, and he gave a wonderful speech about the students, and then introduced Sally, who talked about the Duke of Edinburgh Award scheme. The lights were dimmed and, as Heather Small's song

'Proud' played in the background, we watched an amazing film of Will and his friends and everything they had achieved. To pass the Bronze Award they had to succeed in four different areas. The first was volunteering, and for three months they had created arts and crafts to raise funds for the John Thornton Young Achievers Foundation. The second was physical, and each student had embarked on a fitness programme and had all improved their strength and fitness. The third was the skills section, where each student had a different challenge, and William had been going to Poole College to learn catering. Finally, it was the expeditions, which involved a seventeen-mile walk over two days with overnight camping. They had to learn first aid, erect their own tents, and follow basic map-reading skills to reach their destination.

Not only had each student faced huge challenges and overcome massive personal struggles, my son had done all this and somehow kept it all to himself. Each time I caught Will's eye he looked like the cat that got the cream! Each student was then presented with their certificates, and then they left us with the promise that they'd return with a surprise.

I was fighting back the tears as it was, and then it got even harder. Mr McGill addressed us once more and said, "Now, we have something very special for you. Please give each student a big round of applause as they come back in. Firstly, may I present to you a very special young man who has touched the hearts of us all at Beaucroft. He has an amazing character and has given us all so much fun over the years. We are all going to miss him terribly. Ladies and gentleman, please welcome back, Mr William Matthews."

Will walked back into the room with his shoulders back and a smile from ear-to-ear. He was wearing an academic gown, mortarboard and carrying a scroll as if he was graduating from university. I nearly burst with pride. One by one, each student was introduced; they were all adorned in the same attire and looked incredible. As each proud student took their places again, they played a slide show full of photos of the students throughout all their years at the school. We saw numerous photos of Will we'd never seen over the past thirteen years. It was incredibly emotional, and I was struggling not to cry, when a photo of Will and Daniella appeared on the screen. Will burst into tears. He was sobbing uncontrollably, and when I got up to go and comfort him, he looked through his hands as tears ran through his fingers and said,

"Daddy, I don't want to leave school, I'm going to miss Daniella, I really love her, Dad."

I tried to put my arms around him, but I lost my own battle and had to leave the room. I stood in the boy's toilets, splashing water over my face and trying desperately to pull myself together, but all I could see was Will's tear-stained face. After a couple of minutes, when I felt brave enough, I walked back in to find Daniella comforting Will and most of the room in tears. Somebody had thoughtfully got Daniella from her class and she was cuddling Will and trying to make him feel better. When the presentations were over we went through to the canteen for cream teas, and Daniella's teachers allowed her to miss her last lesson and join us. With each mouthful of scone, they told each other 'I love you hundreds'.

At the end of the day, the students were asked to form in a line out on the sports field for the ceremonial throwing of the mortarboards. We all followed them outside, where there was a professional photographer giving them instructions. When everyone was ready with their own cameras, the photographer shouted, "Right, on the count of three, I want you all to throw your hats as hard as you can. Are you ready? One, two, three!"

They threw them with as much vigour as possible, and many of us got hit by a mortarboard: the photographer had neglected to explain that he meant up! There was a lot of laughing before the students could compose themselves to do it again, and the next time they mastered it. They threw their hats straight and high up into the sky and then gave each other hugs and high-fives. As I watched those amazing young men and women celebrating together, I felt enormously proud of how far Will had come in his time at Beaucroft. I also thought about how much I had changed from the guy who had felt so uncomfortable the first time I visited the school, when I had no idea how to behave around those children. Nobody dreams of having a child with special needs, but don't ever pity me. William has blessed my life in ways I could never have imagined; he is a gift.

The first nineteen years of Will's life have been one hell of an adventure. Despite his limitations, every day he inspires me. He improves the lives of everyone he meets with his honesty, kindness and humour. I look forward to whatever comes next with hope, optimism and a determination, like Will, to always have fun. I know one thing, it'll never be boring. In the words of Heather Small, '*What have you done today to make me feel proud?*' My son makes me proud every single day.

The Extra Bit, The Extra whY?

I am certain that we would all like to change something about ourselves if we could. There are always parts of our physicality that we feel could be better. I am sure that at some point in each of our lives, or even daily, we have looked in a mirror and wished we could improve something about our appearance. If we are really honest, we would admit we could do with improving certain personality traits too. Of course, within reason, we all have the ability to change. Our appearance can be changed dramatically if we make enough effort, and we can all become better human beings if we are open to recognising our faults and are committed to change. But what if it really was possible? What if we actually could make those decisions for our unborn children? Hypothetically, if you could design your own child, what would you choose?

Imagine being an expectant parent and given the freedom to make these choices. After choosing the sex of your child, you'd be allowed to choose from a multitude of physical attributes. The list would be extremely long, and from head to toe you could design what you considered to be the perfect-looking human being. Then, from an even bigger list, you could choose what type of person your child would be. Would you pick high intelligence, outstanding sporting or musical ability? Would you choose drive and determination, or kindness and empathy? Or that they are resistant to illness, healthy and strong? Luckily, you wouldn't have to, as you could choose any quality you wanted. If this was reality, and these were real choices, you would naturally want your child to have every advantage in life.

I don't believe any parent given these choices would choose a physical or mental handicap for their child. No parent wants their child to struggle through life. Why would anyone want their child to suffer? William was born with an extra Y chromosome; his twenty-third pair of chromosomes is genetically different from 99.9% of the male population, and that small difference has altered life for him in immeasurable ways.

As parents we don't always get what we want; but, maybe, we get what we need. Raising William has changed me in ways I'd never imagined possible. I have often heard people say that special children are given to special parents. It's a lovely thought, but I don't think it's true. I believe special children make their parents special. It can be an enormous struggle, and will often push families and relationships to the brink, but with the support of my amazing wife, raising a special child has been the most rewarding experience of my life.